# NO MORE DIRTY LOOKS

# NO MORE DIRTY LOOKS

Siobhan O'Connor

Alexandra Spunt

Da Capo
LIFE
LONG

New York

## Advance Praise for *NO MORE DIRTY LOOKS*

"When it comes to good health, what you put on your skin can be as important as what you put in your mouth. Here's a useful book to help you look better and feel better—without poisoning yourself."

—Eric Schlosser, best-selling author of *Fast Food Nation*

"This book is a wake-up call for all women who think that what you put on your body is not going to hurt you. O'Connor and Spunt offer an in-depth glimpse into the dangers lurking within the beauty industry, in a quick and engaging read that is tough to put down. *No More Dirty Looks* will arm consumers with knowledge, opening their eyes to products they should avoid and safer, healthier alternatives. Every woman I know is getting a copy."

—Kim Barnouin, coauthor of the
#1 *New York Times* best-seller *Skinny Bitch*

"I loved this book! *No More Dirty Looks* is a fabulous and enlightening guide to the cleanest skin, body, and hair care products. It belongs in every woman's library and should be required reading for all skin and hair professionals!"

—Ann Louise Gittleman, Ph.D., *New York Times*
best-selling author of *The Fat Flush Plan*

"*No More Dirty Looks* can save you from many toxic ingredients in cosmetics. Authors O'Connor and Spunt open a wide window to a world where personal care products and safety can co-exist and give you a better result with less pain and danger. The book reads as if the authors are talking with your body—from head to toe."

—Ralph Nader

"As a mom concerned about my own health and that of my child, I consider *No More Dirty Looks* essential reading."

—Jenny McCarthy, author, actress, and activist

The Truth about

Your Beauty Products—

and the Ultimate Guide to

Safe and Clean Cosmetics

Library of Congress Cataloging-in-Publication Data
O'Connor, Siobhan, 1978–
No more dirty looks : the truth about your beauty products—and the ultimate guide to safe and clean cosmetics / Siobhan O'Connor and Alexandra Spunt.
p. cm.
Includes bibliographical references and index.
ISBN 978-0-7382-1396-5 (alk. paper)
1. Cosmetics—Toxicology. 2. Toilet preparations—Toxicology.
I. Spunt, Alexandra, 1978–  I. Title.
RA1270.C65O36 2010
363.19'6—dc22
2010016643

Editorial production by the Book Factory
Design by Jane Raese

First Da Capo Press edition 2010

Published by Da Capo Press
A Member of the Perseus Books Group
www.dacapopress.com

Note: The information in this book is true and complete to the best of our knowledge. This book is intended only as an informative guide for those wishing to know more about health issues. In no way is this book intended to replace, countermand, or conflict with the advice given to you by your own physician. The ultimate decision concerning care should be made between you and your doctor. We strongly recommend you follow his or her advice. Information in this book is general and is offered with no guarantees on the part of the authors or Da Capo Press. The authors and publisher disclaim all liability in connection with the use of this book.

Da Capo Press books are available at special discounts for bulk purchases in the U.S. by corporations, institutions, and other organizations. For more information, please contact the Special Markets Department at the Perseus Books Group, 2300 Chestnut Street, Suite 200, Philadelphia, PA, 19103, or call (800) 810-4145, ext. 5000, or e-mail special.markets@perseusbooks.com.

10 9 8 7 6 5 4 3 2

# Contents

# Contents

# NO
# MORE
# DIRTY
# LOOKS

# Why We're Coming Clean

## THE BLOWOUT

It started with a $400 promise. Get the Brazilian blowout—a fancy new keratin hairstyling treatment—and we'd have perfectly straight, wash-and-go hair for up to two months. This was a couple of years ago, at a time when we both had higher-paying jobs and less level heads. So we went to a posh West Hollywood salon, plopped down into comfy leather chairs, and flipped through tabloids as a mysterious solution was flat-ironed onto our hair. Our eyes watered and the backs of our throats burned, but we barely flinched when the salon offered us protective goggles.

Two teary-eyed hours later, we both had shiny, immaculately straight hair—identical in fact, save for the color. When we'd woken up that morning, our hair could not have been more different: Siobhan's was long, thick, and blonde; Alexandra had a mass of brown curls. Now we looked like Betty and Veronica. As we ran our fingers through our pin-straight locks, we were amazed. It was so . . . pretty. And straight. And stinky.

That evening, over french fries and white wine, we nicknamed our 'dos "toxic molé" for their distinctly unorganic cocoa smell. Instructed to not wash or pin back our hair for forty-eight hours, we would have to get used to it, a sacrifice in the name of delightfully manageable hair.

As the weeks wore on and the stench wore off, our hair was a daily delight. We found the summer humidity tolerable and were happy that our morning routines had been halved. Still, something wasn't sitting right. We're both skeptics by nature and journalists by trade, and this feat of nature started seeming a little, well, unnatural. It would only be a matter of time before something clicked. A matter of time, or a matter of seriously shitty-looking hair, which is what happened next.

The shine had gone matte, our ends were decimated, and we had crowns of flyaways that were most certainly not there before. It was this comedown off the perfect-hair high that fueled our curiosity; we became intent on tracking down just what was in that mysterious solution. That's when the research began and the panic set in. It started with basic Googling (which is never a good idea when you're feeling nervous). We found an article about a woman who'd died days after a similar treatment, asphyxiated by the noxious fumes. As it turns out, the magic ingredient in our lovely Brazilian blowout was not keratin after all.[1] It was formaldehyde.[2]

Before long, we were poring over decades worth of scientific studies and learning the unfamiliar language of chemistry, one fourteen-letter word at a time. At first, it raised more questions than it answered: Why on earth would a beauty treatment contain a known carcinogen? How is that even legal? We considered that it may be an exception to the rule: one rogue company in an otherwise safeguarded industry that was taking advantage of our vanity. But as we dug further, we opened up a Pandora's box of bad news.

We began studying the ingredient lists of our shampoos, our bronzers, our body lotions, and our nail polishes. We noticed a lot of the same words over and over again—propylene glycol, methylparaben, "fragrance"—so we looked them up in medical-research databases. We learned that in addition to the noxious chemicals in our pricey blowouts, there were sketchy ingredients in just about everything we used—from our daily shampooing to our biweekly manicures. We also learned that only 11 percent of the 10,500 ingredients determined by the Food and Drug Administration (FDA) to be in use by the cosmetics industry have been tested for safety by a publicly accountable agency. Of the ones we do know about, some are flat-out dangerous to our health, others are questionable at best, and most are doing almost nothing to improve the quality, feel, and health of our skin and hair.[3] So not only are these products wreaking some unspeakable havoc on our bodies, they're also making us look *worse*.

*What a drag*, we thought. Like most women, we had an arsenal of products we swore by. We'd given these brands our trust (and our money) for years. But then something incredible happened. As we started switching to clean beauty products, we began to feel and see a difference in our appearances. And it was a good difference. Our skin was clearer, our hair calmed down—we even smelled better once we found a decent natural deodorant.

It makes sense: the bottom line for most businesses is just that—the bottom line. Large cosmetics companies have huge product runs that must be able to withstand years on the shelf and remain stable in all kinds of climates and conditions. This kind of manufacturing is not always going to be about supplying you with the highest-quality, most beautifying ingredients for your buck. So they pad their products with cheap, widely accepted fillers, and spend the big coin on marketing campaigns.

But it's not as though they don't know the science. They've read the same reports we have, and then some. So why are they selling us these things? In the words of one industry scientist whose employer charges $250 for a 2-ounce pot of face cream, "Because we can."

## OUTSIDE IN

Skin is a moody organ, finicky about what it lets in and what it keeps out. Yes, it is a protective layer, which is why when you spill water on yourself, you don't melt like the Wicked Witch of the West. At the same time, our dermis *does* let in lots of other things we put on it—as much as 60 percent, by some accounts.[4]

If you've ever tried to quit smoking, you may be familiar with the nicotine patch. If you were lucky, it gave you Technicolor dreams and curbed your cigarette cravings by supplying you with a steady flow of nicotine. The patch can do that thanks to transdermal absorption, an effective way of getting all kinds of things right into your bloodstream. Skin is a popular delivery route for many medications, precisely because it's so direct. Think about that. Now think about how much you put on your skin, and how often.

You probably bathe daily. Every other day, sometimes? Fair enough; us, too. But every time we decide we want to wash, plump, moisturize, nourish, shine, buff, soften, bronze, and otherwise play around with how we look and feel, we are reaching for a bottle whose contents are largely a mystery. That's not because we're all idiots; that's the way the cosmetics industry has set it up. They will boast about one or two ingredients in their ads—usually the natural ones—while obscuring the bulk of the ingredients in four-point font in a barely contrasting color on the edge of the bottle. And yet ingredient lists are the most transparent thing these companies provide us.

Now consider that many of us use up to twenty products a day, from body wash to mascara, and everything in between. With each product containing anywhere from twenty to fifty or more ingredients—not to mention artificial fragrance, which we'll get to—that's up to one thousand chemicals we're exposing ourselves to every single day, sometimes twice a day, without having a clue what these things are, not to mention how they interact together in the bottle and on our bodies.

Meanwhile, no independent authority or government agency is monitoring what cosmetics companies put in our products. The FDA's Office of Cosmetics and Colors has a couple of rules in place, and it likes to say it regulates the industry, but a closer look reveals that the beauty business is, in fact, almost entirely self-regulated. That isn't to say that no safety testing is being done; it's just that it's being done almost exclusively by the cosmetics companies themselves. It's a system whose checks and balances are woefully inadequate, allowing for the widespread use of some pretty questionable substances.

That's because the cosmetics laws in the United States haven't really changed since 1938. Since then, cosmetics have gotten incredibly sophisticated and have exploded into a $35 billion industry. Unchecked business, massive profits, and outdated laws: remind you of any other industries?

## WHERE THIS BOOK COMES IN

If cruising government websites, poring over toxicological data, and performing science experiments on your face isn't your idea of fun, don't worry—because it's ours. We've spent thousands of hours digging up all kinds of things the beauty industry doesn't want you to know, and now we're going to share them with you. We're also going to take a good hard look at the ingredients in our everyday products, offer answers to all your pesky beauty problems, and show you how your current cosmetics might be contributing to them. Then (and this is the fun part), we will help you choose better, safer beauty products and learn easy do-it-yourself recipes you'll love—these will have you looking, feeling, and smelling better in no time.

We've personally tried everything that we recommend in this book, and then some. Each product and recipe meets our standards in terms of quality, safety, and vanity—and we're a picky pair. We also have temperamental skin, care about aging, worry about the environmental footprint of our products, and like to look our best. But fear not: we're not going to force you to chuck your favorite night-out lipstick or tell you to give up highlights forever. We just want to help you minimize your health risks and make smarter, easier beauty choices.

To ease you through your transition, we have arranged our chapters by body part. We will look at the ingredients used in most products, walk you through the research, explore the health concerns associated with them, and then help you deepen your understanding of how your body works. Each chapter also contains easy-to-follow how-tos, a comprehensive guide of the best products out there—and some pot shots at the companies selling us all those crappy potions.

## RESISTING THE URGE TO BE
## TOTAL CONSPIRACY-THEORIST WACKJOBS

Certainly, the question keeps popping up in our minds. If some cosmetics ingredients are dangerous—or at least not proven to be safe—then why on earth would a company use them? Are they trying to make us sick? Is it a great breast-cancer conspiracy? Not really. "Unlike the cigarette companies," says Dr. Mitchell A. Kline, a top New York City dermatologist and researcher, "which had intent to obscure the medical studies, I don't think these companies have intent. But I do think they are turning a blind eye. It has washed over them, and the inertia has carried them along."

But why has nothing been done about it? As Dr. Michael DiBartolomeis, a toxicologist and the chief of the California Safe Cosmetics Program, says, "What regulatory agencies have to do is prove something is bad—so instead of manufacturers proving something is safe, it's the other way around. It's perfectly set up to allow lots of bad things out into the market."

Then there's the financial angle. We know that certain ingredients are super-cheap, and that they can extend the life of a product for years. We also know that *not* reformulating products is way easier, and a lot less expensive, than recalling and reformulating. And at the end of the day, if we get sick in twenty years, it'll be really hard for anyone to prove it's because we used some face cream our whole life. So it's a little tricky.

We're not suggesting that the cosmetics industry is deliberately poisoning us. But research about dozens of questionable ingredients is mounting, and it's only going to become harder for them to ignore it. Concern about BPA, and phthalates more broadly, has garnered attention in the pages of leading newspapers and magazines, and influential medical organizations are beginning to release strongly worded statements about how certain chemicals can adversely affect our bodies. A sea change is upon us, but resistance persists. As author and activist Stacy Malkan puts it, "The science we have on concerns about chronic, low-dose chemical exposure and the links to disease is all relatively new information. Not brand new—anyone paying attention knows about this. But there really is an entrenched belief that low-dose chemical exposure is okay. I think it's hard for people after thirty years of a career to admit or acknowledge that things are entirely different from what they were taught. The other part of it, of course, is a corporate resistance to change that would cost time and money."

Bingo. As Kline puts it, "It all has to come down to money. These are people who make billions of dollars selling products. It's very difficult to beat them and their researchers by changing the law, which requires lobbying and a lot of money."

That leaves us with some uncomfortable questions and unsatisfying answers. So allow us to introduce to you our "why bother" clause. As in, "If you can't be sure a product is safe—and it's not doing your looks any favors—why bother using it?" It's our mantra. We hope it'll be yours, too.

# 2

# The Regulation Game

## Inside the Wild West of the Beauty Industry

Understanding how the beauty industry works is an essential part of the larger conversation we're tackling here. While it may be boring to some, we find it strangely fascinating to see just how broken the system is. And to even think about changing it, we need to come from an informed place. So no yawning.

That said, if policy talk causes your eyes to glaze over, here are our *CliffsNotes*: no government agency has your back here. Companies can and do use pretty much anything they like in their products, because that's how the laws are written. As a result, cosmetics companies—yes, even the fancy ones—tend to load up their products with cheap, mass-produced, and sometimes unsafe ingredients. And while they like to point to the FDA whenever anyone questions how safe their products are, the FDA's rules about cosmetics barely even exist, and the ones that do aren't readily enforced. Sure, companies test their products before they put them to market; it's bad for business when people have noticeable adverse reactions. But the rub is that these companies aren't legally bound to do so. Why? Because the industry is, for all intents and purposes, a profit-focused, self-policed free-for-all.

Parts of the world have kept pace with the science and have adjusted their cosmetics laws accordingly. Canada, while similarly lax, shows encouraging signs that its ear is to the ground for chemicals of concern. Health Canada provides a hot list of restricted ingredients, but mostly it follows the FDA's lead and relies largely on the safety data produced by the American product council—an industry umbrella that represents most of the brands you know by name.[1] The European Union, meanwhile, has been on this stuff for years, banning a whopping one-thousand-plus ingredients that are still widely used in most of the products you find at the pharmacy. While American companies do reformulate for Europe, they do not elsewhere—and even the stricter E.U. laws have holes in them. With more than ten thousand chemicals in use by the cosmetics industry, everyone can stand to learn more about these products.

For the United States, here are the facts at a glance:

- The FDA does not test everyday personal-care products for safety before they hit the market.
- The FDA does not require companies to provide safety data about its products.
- If a product is found to be unsafe, the FDA cannot easily force a company to recall it.
- Most of the "safety" testing being done is focused on short-term reactions, such as rashes, and is conducted by the corporations that sell the products.
- No one knows the long-term effects of many of the chemicals used.

- Cosmetics companies can use almost any ingredient under the sun, without any oversight.
- Europe has banned more than one thousand ingredients for use in personal-care products. The United States has banned nine.
- Some ingredients can migrate into body tissue and do not leave the body right away.
- Leading public health experts say there is no such thing as a "safe" dosage of a carcinogen, yet several are still used in very common personal care products.
- Many toxic chemicals make it into your beauty products as byproducts and are therefore not listed on labels.
- The fragrance industry is protected under trade secret laws, which means the ingredients are not listed on labels at all.

That's the short version; the long version is even juicier. But first, meet Betty Bridges, a registered nurse whose experience will help put some of these facts into perspective.

## ONE WOMAN'S STORY

Betty Bridges was at work when the first attack hit. It was 1988, and she was performing her routine duties at the health clinic when, all of a sudden, she couldn't breathe. "I just could not get any air in," she says now. But when she ran outside, the feeling was gone.

The clinic had recently changed its brand of all-purpose cleaner, and she quickly figured out that every time she came near it, her lungs would constrict. I must be allergic to something in it, she thought. But when she compared the ingredients between the old cleaner and the new one, the only difference she noticed was that the new one contained "fragrance."

Before long, the attacks began to hit more frequently. It wasn't just cleaners triggering the reaction, but perfumes, detergents—even deodorant. She figured her reactions must be caused by a fairly common ingredient—it couldn't be that hard to isolate. Oh, but it could. Due to consumer-unfriendly trade-secret laws and the fact that any one fragrance can contain *hundreds* of different chemicals, identifying the offending ingredient would take Bridges eight years.

Noting that she reacted to one kind of clothing detergent and not another from the same brand, Bridges called up the manufacturer thinking they might be of assistance. It wasn't as easy as that, though. She was told they wouldn't be able to help her—that their formula was proprietary.

And thanks to laws that protect companies from having to give up ingredient lists for their fragrances (lest someone steal their secret formulas), that detergent manufacturer was well within its rights to tell her to buzz off.

But she stayed on the case. By 1995, her life had been severely impacted by her allergy. She'd left her job as a nurse, working instead at her husband's cabinet shop where she could avoid scents that triggered her reactions. "But if a guy came in wearing cologne," she says with a laugh, "I would run to the back."

Around that time, she began posting online about her condition and reading everything she could. Finally, she found a sympathetic fragrance chemist who offered to help. He instructed her to do some controlled testing with several products. Once she narrowed it down, he sent her four pure chemical samples that he suspected might be triggering her reactions, which she then took to her doctor's office. Lo and behold, when her doctor assessed her breath after inhaling one of the chemicals, they finally had their answer. It is called, mysteriously, CAS No. 122-40-7. Also known as *amyl cinnamal*, CAS No. 122-40-7 is a floral-smelling liquid used in all kinds of detergents, shampoos, and bath products—which is why Bridges had trouble getting away from the stuff.[2]

Bridges channeled her frustration into even more research—most of it sourced directly from the fragrance industry. She poured her findings into an exhaustive website, fpinva.org, and became a fragrance-industry watchdog of sorts. She teamed up with another activist, Barb Wilkie, and together they sent a popular perfume they'd been hearing complaints about to a fragrance analysis lab in New York.[3] "Forty-two chemicals were identified," Bridges says, "but when I went to research the first ingredient listed [Iso E Super], it had very little [safety] data available. And despite this, the product carried no warning label." Among the other chemicals identified were endocrine disruptors and suspected carcinogens.[4]

With the help of the Environmental Health Network of California, Bridges and Wilkie petitioned the FDA in 1999 to declare the product misbranded. They also say they produced about one thousand letters of support. So far, the FDA has taken no action.

## MEET THE FDA

You're going to hear the FDA mentioned pretty frequently here, and not because we have such a rage on for them (though we'll certainly take a few jabs where they're warranted). It's just that most of us have never had a clear understanding of what they do or, as in the case of cosmetics, don't do.

If you're like us, you probably assume that the FDA's Office of Cosmetics and Colors regulates your beauty products in some way or another. You figure that your lipstick, your shampoo, and your stretch mark cream have all been tested and approved by some public health agency that says, "Yup, this is safe." You also might imagine that there are loads of ingredients that companies can't use because they're unsafe or untested, and won't use because they're disgusting—things like formaldehyde and crushed beetles.

See, that's what would make sense. But alas, in this upside-down world, 'tis not the case (not even the part about bugs, though starting in 2011 companies will have to list them as cochineal or carmine on the label).[5] Instead, the FDA is essentially a cosmetics regulation figurehead. It seems powerful, and the cosmetics companies like to say they are in compliance with FDA regulations, but that agency doesn't even have the authority to give pre-market approval of finished products. So what exactly are these companies "complying" with? Not a whole lot.

The FDA can't require manufacturers to send in lists of the ingredients they're using. And while the European Union has banned more than one thousand ingredients for use in cosmetics, the FDA has banned or restricted only nine.[6] Then, when something goes wrong—like a string of allergic reactions or some other unintended effect—the FDA can't even force a recall of a cosmetic. Instead, the agency can recommend a recall to the company that makes the product. And if said company doesn't play nice, and the FDA has registered public complaints about a certain product, it can take them to court.[7] As you can probably guess, that doesn't happen all that often.

Sounds insane, but think about it: you know how when you go to the farmers market, there's always a nice hippie chick selling soaps she made in her kitchen? That's a decent (if loose) comparison to how the beauty giants operate. She, like the major cosmetics corporations, doesn't have to tell the FDA who she is, what's in the stuff she's selling, nor must she report it if someone's skin turns blue after using her lotion.[8]

When this finally sank in, it really burned us up, especially since none of it is actually a secret. Anyone who's ventured as far as the FDA's website knows as much. It's all written there in plain language. But just because the information is publicly available does not mean people know about it or, more important, that it makes any sense.

Without regulatory safeguards in place, our health is in the hands of a couple of cosmetics-industry trade organizations, both of which have financial ties to the beauty business. You'll get to know them in a second, but understand that they are large, well funded, and incredibly influential. (One scientist we spoke to likened them to the Mafia, another to the lobbyists for Big Tobacco in its heyday.) These trade groups insist they work with impartial experts who have public safety in mind, and that may very well be true. But they also spend a lot of time and money lobbying against government regulation of personal-care products.

For the record, we're not a couple of commie government-control cheerleaders. In fact, more stringent oversight might put significant strain on some brands we know and love (not to mention the soap lady at the farmers market). It would cost quite a chunk of change and time and manpower to jump through federal hoops providing toxicological data, complying with quality control regulations, and so on. Our hunch, though, is that folks who care about your safety would do it, and they would do it with a smile on their face. Because it's their opinion, and ours, that anything that gets inside your body—prescription drugs, food, and ingredients in almost all cosmetics—should come with the reassurance that it is safe. And if it's not, we should be given a clear sense of the risks involved. Until then, combing ingredient lists on labels and asking good questions is your best move (more about how to do this in Chapter 3). First, though . . .

## A LITTLE HISTORY

One hundred years ago, consumables, drugs, and cosmetics were sort of a free-for-all. It sounds kind of fun (Cocaine for breakfast! Aphrodisiacs for dinner!), but people were getting sick, and the public was starting to panic. In 1906, the feds stepped in. The Food and Drug Act of 1906 was the first major law of its kind, and though it didn't cover cosmetics, it did put limits on what the food and drug industries could get away with.[9] The act initiated the process of governments protecting our health from companies trying to make a quick buck. It dealt mostly with labeling regulations and the use of chemical additives in foods, so like, if you say it's beef, it better not be horsemeat, and it better not have poisonous preservatives in it.[10]

That act also showed that when it comes to getting laws changed, the squeaky wheel gets the grease. The law was ratified, thanks in large part to growing pressure from Bureau of Chemistry chief Harvey Washington Wiley and shit disturbers like Upton Sinclair, both of whose research was causing quite the stir among consumers. (Sinclair's 1906 novel, *The Jungle*, was a harsh indictment of the meatpacking industry, and after the book came out, meat sales plummeted. It spawned a President Roosevelt–backed investigation into the business, and eventually practices changed. The book is considered a major impetus to the Food and Drug Act's passing.)[11]

But while that act got the ball rolling, it also left a lot of room for enterprising businesses. In the next few decades, all kinds of crazy products made it to market, including a growing number of promise-filled and problematic cosmetics. Exhibit A: Lash Lure, a permanent mascara that caused blindness, severe disfiguration, and at least one death.[12] Exhibit B: Kormelu, a depilatory cream laced with carcinogenic rat poison.[13]

It wasn't until 1930 that the Bureau of Chemistry and other governing bodies got reshuffled and officially became the FDA. From the get-go, the FDA faced mounting pressure to extend its jurisdiction to cover cosmetics. Word was out that the industry was the Wild West, and in the early 1930s, the *New Republic* published several essays about the dangers of unregulated beauty products.[14] The American Medical Association, too, was on the bandwagon.[15] Within a few years, the FDA as we know it now took shape.

Finally, a new bill was sponsored. This one included cosmetics and sought to overhaul existing food and drug regulation as well, but it took a national tragedy for it to garner real attention: in 1937, more than one hundred people died, including many children, after ingesting a pediatric "miracle" drug that turned out to contain an ingredient closely related to antifreeze. The following year, the revised 1938 Food, Drug, and Cosmetic Act passed, putting cosmetics under federal regulation for the first time.

The 1938 act defined what cosmetics are, how they should be labeled, and said that decaying, harmful, and poisonous substances can't be used in them.[16] (It stopped short of specifics, though.) It excluded soap and hair dyes from this already limited scope, and has remained largely unchanged ever since.

Among the small changes since 1938 was the 1960 Color Additive Amendment, which was enacted due to growing concern about dyes in food and—you guessed it—beauty products. That amendment banned the use of colors shown to cause cancer in humans or animals, and required pre-market approval of color additives by the FDA.[17] Later that decade, a labeling act passed saying that any cosmetics that move across state borders (which in modern times means basically all of them) must be honestly labeled.[18]

In 1973, things got interesting: a Democratic senator from Missouri, Thomas Eagleton, proposed a bill that, had it passed, would have rendered this whole conversation moot. He wanted the FDA to begin conducting pre-market clearance of cosmetics, wanted full ingredient disclosure, wanted cosmetics companies to register with the FDA, felt that complaint-filing should be streamlined, and so on.[19] It would have meant a massive shift and would have addressed a lot of the concerns activists and consumers still hold today. But the cosmetic industry trade organization—the one that claims to have our safety in mind—fought hard against it and won. It won again in 1988 when Ron Wyden, a Democrat from Oregon, proposed a similar bill.[20] That one, obviously, didn't go anywhere, either.

## WHERE WE ARE TODAY

Welcome to today. If you think we're skipping over a few decades to save you the boring history lesson, you're mistaken. Sure, some things changed here and there, some papers were pushed around, but the FDA's Cosmetics and Colors Office operates pretty much the same way it always has, because that's all the law will permit it to do. The FDA says that companies are required to provide adequate proof of a product's safety, and that if they can't, they have to have a label on it saying so. We don't know about you, but we've never seen a product label at Sephora that says "Warning: The safety of this product has not been determined," although many probably should.

In the meantime, cosmetics have gotten incredibly sophisticated. Your grandma's cold cream isn't the anti-aging silver bullet anymore. Now it's products with "nanoparticles," promises of "bioperformance," and other sciencey terms that blur the line between cosmetics and drugs (and push the limits of the English language, too). Industry people like to call them "cosmeceuticals," a cute hybrid term that is not recognized by the FDA as having any legal definition, so it can mean anything the beauty companies want it to mean.[21] We're not talking about your prescription Retin-A here, which contains a regulated drug. We're talking about the anti-wrinkle aisle at the pharmacy or department store, with all its pretty bottles and outrageous promises. Some of their druglike ingredients and therapeutic druglike claims should certainly merit their being treated as drugs under the law. Because guess what? Drugs *do* need to be assessed by the FDA before they hit the market. Yet not your fancy wrinkle cream.

If any of this sounds like bullshit, we encourage you to take five minutes to Google "FDA" and "cosmetics" and read the official government literature yourself. You'll find that "with the exception of color additives and a few prohibited ingredients, a cosmetics manufacturer may, on his own responsibility, use *essentially any raw material* as a cosmetics ingredient and market the product without approval" (emphasis ours). It's all written in plain English. There's even an easy-to-read FAQ.

Turns out, we're not the only ones who think the laws are a little out of date. In the first decade of the twenty-first century, consumer advocacy groups such as the Environmental Working Group and their Campaign for Safe Cosmetics, Teens Turning Green, a handful of politicians, public health researchers, and journalists have been working overtime to change these outdated laws and/or educate consumers. In 2009, U.S. Representative Jan Schakowsky told the *Washington Post*: "The fact that we are bathing our kids in products contaminated with carcinogens shows how woefully out of date our cosmetics laws are and how urgently they need to be updated. . . . The science has moved forward; now the FDA needs to catch up and be given the authority to protect the health of Americans."

We agree with her. But a lot would have to change. The Cosmetics and Colors Office at the FDA is only as powerful as Congress makes it. In 2009, the FDA's cosmetics office had an annual allowance of $5.5 million[22]—less than 0.2 percent of the FDA's total annual budget. The office also has only about thirty people on its staff.[23] With the laws set up as they are, and with those limited resources, there's a lot more they can't do, than can.

We would love to see Congress give the FDA the go-ahead to reinvent itself. But for that to happen, it's going to take a major shift in public opinion and spending and a lot of pressure on lawmakers to create policy change. That's why we need you to suffer through a couple more pages of this stuff. Because when you begin to proselytize about this to your friends and family, to your boyfriends, and to the stranger on the subway, we don't want you to be written off as some ill-informed reactionary dork. We want you armed and dangerous with the two most convincing weapons: (1) stone cold facts, and (2) a hotter you. We're gonna get to the latter soon. *Promise.*

## INSIDE THE BEAUTY BUSINESS

The Personal Care Product Council (PCPC) is the big, huge, powerful industry group that represents more than six hundred cosmetics companies, which together account for almost all the products on shelves nationwide. The council has been around in some form or another since the late 1800s, and its member list is a who's-who of the beauty biz. Check out the stuff in your bathroom and most of it probably comes from one of its members. L'Oréal? Check. Avon? Check. Elizabeth Arden, Chanel, Estée Lauder, Philosophy, Johnson & Johnson's, Clarins, Revlon, Mary Kay, Colgate? Check.

The PCPC, which used to be called the CFTA (for clarity, though, we're going to refer to them as the PCPC going forward), is made up of lobbyists, scientists, policy experts, public-relations folks, and a guy who used to head up the FDA's cosmetics department. On its website is the claim that it is the "voice on scientific, legal, regulatory, legislative, and international issues for the personal care product industry."[24] That sums it up pretty well. It's also the group that powers up the PR machine when someone says cosmetics might not be so good for you.

It makes sense. Bad press is bad for business, and together, its member companies are estimated to represent 80 percent of the products sold in the United States.[25] That's tens of billions of dollars worth of business. The council also prides itself on its rigorous science, its consumer website that looks an awful lot like the Campaign for Safe Cosmetics' (but without the comprehensive information), and its safety assessments, done through the Cosmetics Ingredient Review (CIR). CIR is a PCPC-funded panel of chemists and medical experts that assesses ingredients for safety. We know what you're thinking: "Thank god *someone* is testing these things." Right? Not so fast.

Another thing the PCPC does is lobby. If experience begets expertise, then the PCPC should be a pro by now, since the group had its first lobbying coup in 1919, when Prohibition threatened to imperil toiletries containing alcohol. (Don't worry, though, they had the wording changed so that business could continue as usual.)[26] It also did well in the 1970s, when proregulation sentiment was heating up, thanks to the Eagleton bill. The trade organization handled the matter dexterously, and in the end, it ended up working with the FDA to enact a new regulation that said companies must be able to substantiate their safety claims or else have a warning on the product—a vague and poorly enforced edict, and a far cry from the oversight Eagleton was after.

The PCPC has always wielded a lot of power, and that couldn't be truer today. In the second quarter of 2008, it spent a comparatively meager half a million dollars lobbying against proposed regulations on cosmetics. That same year, it also arranged meetings between 150 legislators and industry representatives.[27] We're educated-guessing here, but we assume that means industry executives telling politicians how safe cosmetics are, and that lawmakers should go ahead and back off. That same year, twenty-two states considered—and ultimately did *not* pass—legislation related to labeling, safety, and ingredient-reporting.[28] The PCPC highlighted that as an accomplishment in its annual report.

Why does the PCPC need to lobby at all? Every controversial business does it. In 2009, one of the largest oil companies in the world was still paying lobbyists to push ideas that global-warming is a sham. Now, the tides are turning on cosmetics, too, and the industry is very much aware of it. It has been talking for years in its annual reports about "rumors and misinformation" spreading on the Internet, about "attacks" by activists, and about "anti-cosmetics" legislation in states such as California. As such, the PCPC has pledged to continue to reach out to politicians, legislators, thought leaders, and influencers, presumably to make sure they don't get any crazy ideas, either.

Oh, and us. Don't forget us. Cosmetics companies want us to love them and think nice things about them, too, so they hire our favorite celebrities to pose with their perfume, they have philanthropic efforts where they give away makeup to breast cancer patients, they sponsor community events, they donate money to research, and they advertise to us in our magazines.

See, they're super good at what they do. That's why in addition to having scientists on their staffs formulating and testing their products, they also lean on the Cosmetic Ingredient Review (CIR)—a panel that assesses safety on the industry's behalf. Put on your lab coats, ladies. Time to meet some scientists.

## A SCIENTIFIC SAFEGUARD?

Recall, if you will, how in the 1970s, politicians and consumers were getting all worked up about the need for cosmetics regulation. Well, around then, the trade organization threw the FDA a bone and created its very own panel of safety experts. Founded in 1976, the Cosmetics Ingredient Review is made up of nine voting members who give the PCPC recommendations on different ingredients.[29] It's also what the PCPC brings up when questions arise about a lack of regulation in the business, as if to say, "How could these be unsafe? Our independent panel of world-class experts works extremely hard to assess the safety of the ingredients we use." And they would know how hard the CIR works, of course, because they're the ones signing their paychecks.[30]

The CIR does not itself test ingredients or products, though. Instead, its panel reviews scientific research on high-priority ingredients, then meets four times a year to discuss the findings. These meetings are often open to other people, too—not just the nine voting members. At a March 2009 meeting, for example, there were reps from Unilever, Shiseido, L'Oréal, the FDA, and the PCPC.[31]

At these meetings, the CIR expert panel will discuss what it has found. If there is not enough data, it'll say so and recommend that more tests be done. If there is enough data, the panel debates, discusses, and votes on the findings, and a final report is generated. That report gives safety recommendations. For example: Beauty Ingredient is safe the way it's currently used; Beauty Ingredient is unsafe the way it's currently used; or Beauty Ingredient is safe in concentrations up to X percent. Those reports then go to the PCPC, the FDA's Cosmetics office, and others.

Between 1976 and 2008, the CIR assessed 1,468 ingredients for safety, all of which are listed in a Quick Reference Table on its website. That's 11 percent of the ingredients listed in the cosmetic-ingredient dictionary that the PCPC uses.[32] The PCPC insists that list is much longer than the list of chemicals it actually uses. (To which we say, "It's *your* dictionary, guys. We're just doing the math.") To this day, only nine ingredients have been deemed unsafe for use in cosmetics; the vast majority is deemed safe as used or safe with restrictions.[33] Call us crazy, but that seems statistically fishy. To us, that means either the cosmetics companies are doing a bang-up job using only truly safe ingredients, or that the CIR's criteria for calling an ingredient safe are a little loose.

It's worth looking at what happens when the CIR *does* recommend specific limits on ingredients in beauty products. In a 2007 letter from Massachusetts Senator John Kerry (yes, that John Kerry) to the FDA, he cited a 2004 study by the Environmental Working Group (EWG) that found *hundreds* of products on the market in the United States *in violation of CIR safety recommendations.*[34] Two years before that, someone from the FDA sent a strongly worded letter to the PCPC about that same study, saying it was considering "compliance action."[35] None was taken.

## INSIDE THE FRAGRANCE BUSINESS

Before we dive in, don't think for a second that if you don't wear perfume that this next bit does not apply to you. "Fragrance" is listed as a single ingredient on the labels of just about everything you use. Because of trade-secret laws, however, that one word alone can represent as many as several hundred additional chemicals that do not need to be listed on labels.[36] As you can imagine, this represents a unique obstacle for those of us trying to screen our products for dangerous substances.

Trying to find answers about how the fragrance industry operates is harder than getting a Mason to teach you their secret handshake. Here's why: first, the laws protect them from having to tell you what they're using. Second, that "fragrance" in your body lotion is rarely made by the company that sells you that body lotion. Instead, it is manufactured by independent fragrance houses whose names you almost certainly do not know, and which you would have trouble tracking down if you wanted to. These houses have the unique job of producing the ingredient compounds that make your products smell like roses (or peaches, or apples, or anything else under the sun). So not only do you not know what's in there, the company selling it to you might not, either.

Fragrance is essentially a whole other industry, with its own rules and lobbyists and trade groups with expert panels. One of those is the Research Institute for Fragrance Materials (RIFM), which was founded in 1966 by the fragrance industry to evaluate the safety of its ingredients.[37] RIFM is considered the "scientific arm" of the fragrance trade organization, and its expert panel is made up of scientists and medical professionals who function much like the CIR does for the cosmetics business.[38] It's the organization responsible for evaluating the safety of the chemicals used industry-wide. So it looks over available data, agrees on safety recommendations, and submits its findings to the International Fragrance Association (IFRA) (the trade organization that represents the industry) for review. It is this group—not the one doing safety assessments—that then establishes guidelines for the industry. While these guidelines aren't enforceable by law, fragrance manufacturers are expected to abide by them. What happens if they don't? Their name is listed on IFRA's website as "non-IFRA compliant." This happens only if they are a member of the trade organization to begin with, though.[39] And you probably haven't heard of this company or to whom they supply.

When you consider how many chemicals go into making any single smell, and then you consider the fact that these smells are often formulated by fragrance manufacturers, you begin to wonder how that works from a safety perspective. How much does that body-lotion company know about the fragrances it's buying? When we spoke to RIFM, they told us that depends on the relationship between the supplier and the company, adding that, most of the time, the companies know what they're using. Dr. Dave Hobson, an industry toxicologist, doesn't seem to think that is the case. "Because of the proprietary and trade-secret nature of fragrances," he says, "there's going to be limited or no information provided on the chemical substances they are composed of."

If you're starting to think that this system lacks the proper checks and balances to guarantee your safety, you're not alone. Betty Bridges, that same registered nurse with a serious fragrance allergy, founded the Fragrance Product Information Page for just that reason. Her website aims to deliver accurate information about the chemicals used in the fragrances and their health risks. According to her research, RIFM has major holes in its safety data, including a whole bunch of chemicals with little to no information at all.

When we asked RIFM how many of the chemicals used in fragrance it had safety data on, we were told that of the estimated 2,300 chemicals used, they have summaries of data on about 1,100, thanks to a "new evaluation process." Combine that with data from their old evaluation process, and, we were told, somewhere between 70 to 80 percent of the chemicals are covered.

This raises a few obvious questions: What about the other 20 to 30 percent? And were these chemicals tested for skin reactions, such as rashes? Or were they tested for the effects of long-term exposure? Finally, what happens when these chemicals are used together? Our simple questions did not provide us with the kind of concrete answers one would hope for, especially when you consider some of the skeletons in the industry's closet.

Back in the 1970s a synthetic musk called AETT was a common ingredient in perfume, soaps, and detergent. It had been in use for more than twenty years before researchers discovered that repeated exposure to the stuff was turning rats blue. It wasn't just their skin, either, though that was the tip-off—their brains, spinal cords, and nerves were blue, proving that the ingredient was able to migrate into body tissue. AETT was causing severe neurological damage to these rats, and the discovery led to the industry's voluntary withdrawal of the chemical from use.[40] But between the discovery of the bluing in 1975, and 1978, when it was removed from use, no recalls or public announcements were made.

That was then. Not a whole lot has changed, but thanks to consumers' increased focus on transparency, and thanks to the Internet, things might begin moving in the right direction.

As for Betty Bridges—her story has somewhat of a happy ending. The chemical she reacts to is one of the twenty-four for which Europe now requires a warning label. Since then, the industry at large has been slowly phasing out good old CAS No. 122-40-7. As a result, Bridges gets to breathe a little more easily now.

# 3

## Dirty Ingredients

Grab your loupe, because it's time to read the fine print on all those little bottles that crowd your bathroom. In this chapter we're going to show you how to read your cosmetics labels in the same way you would your box of cereal. If you're the kind of person who'd rather just get a list from the nutritionist and chow down, you're out of luck. This is important stuff: it will help answer burning questions like "Do I need to throw out my value-pack of bar soap?" "What are phthalates, and why should I care?" and "Could my lipstick give my unborn child brain damage?"

### MEET YOUR FRIENDLY NEIGHBORHOOD CHEMICALS

Look no further than the ads in your favorite women's magazine and you'll know awareness about cosmetics ingredients is on the rise. All of a sudden it's "sulfate-free" this and "paraben-free" that. As consumers get savvier, so do cosmetics companies. In response to the chatter, many companies are reformulating to omit one or two of the ingredients that have become buzzwords, and then they mount advertising campaigns bragging about it. That is what we call marketing—but leaving out one ingredient and replacing it with a lesser-known or chemically similar substitute is not necessarily what we call clean. Neither is boasting about its absence when your products are packed with a dozen other dirty chemicals.

But don't just take our word for it. To help you understand why that's not quite good enough, we're going to look at roughly twenty widely used ingredients or byproducts that have some not-so-hot scientific data published about them. We'll also explain how to find them on your product labels and hear from experts about why you might want to stay away.

This list is by no means exhaustive (but for quick reference, and a more comprehensive list, check the appendix). As you now understand from the last chapter, between trade secrets, lobbying, incomplete ingredient lists, and data gaps, it would be virtually impossible to present you with a complete list. Instead, we've chosen the most common ones that are used in a mind-boggling range of products, many of which beg questions like, "Why the hell does my $100 under-eye cream contain the same crap as my $6 conditioner?"

Keep in mind that when it comes to science, you're never going to get hard and fast answers (trust us, we've tried). There are so many factors to consider, and proving that your shampoo is the cause of your psoriasis or, worse, your liver damage, is extremely difficult. But just because organs aren't always turning blue does not mean that some of these chemicals aren't taking long-term tolls on our health. These chemicals tax our already-burdened bodies.

Of course, it is difficult to prove that some of these ingredients are making us sick. Here's why: let's say that Chemical X is patch-tested on some mice. Aside from a few rashes, X seems to have no other deleterious effects. However, when X is injected into the mice in larger doses, it causes severe liver damage. Based on that study, recommendations will be made about the percentage of X that can be used in a product. But what would happen if the mice were patch-tested with X every day for fifteen years? Would they have liver damage then? Something else? Does Chemical X stay in their bodies and build up over time (a process known as "bioaccumulation")? And even if it doesn't, how much strain is it putting on the body? What if it reacts badly with another chemical in the same product, creating an altogether new set of reactions?

See, you're not going to find *proof* that your hair spray causes birth defects. There may be strong scientific links but not conclusive evidence. The problem is that this disconcerting data exists, everyone in the scientific and cosmetics communities has read it, and very little is being done about it.

## MEET SOME EXPERTS

The science that looks at how living organisms are affected by chemicals is toxicology. Toxicologists are a divided bunch when it comes to this stuff, and determining what is safe and what is not is far from an exact science. On one side you find someone like Dr. Dave Hobson, a toxicologist who works as an independent consultant for several major cosmetics companies. Hobson takes human safety seriously; it's his job. According to him, the "fundamental maxim in the science of toxicology, is this: the dosage makes the poison." This is the mantra of the cosmetics industry; we heard it a lot when we were writing this book. It means that in small amounts, these ingredients are considered safe.

On the other side of the ring are toxicologists like Dr. Michael DiBartolomeis from the California Department of Public Health. "I can't tell you if there is any safe level for any carcinogen," he says. He does not think the risk-based approach is adequate. "If I hear someone talk about dose one more time, I might throw up. It's just not that simple. If it were, you wouldn't have so many toxicologists arguing about it."

We also spoke with Dr. Joseph A. Schwarcz. This McGill University chemist is the author of several books and articles about chemicals we encounter in our everyday lives. He's devoted most of his career to making science understandable to lay folk. While he certainly seems to lean toward the risk-based assessment of chemical exposure, when we pressed him about possible consequences of long-term exposure to such a wide variety of chemicals (and in so many combinations), he leveled with us: "Those are very reasonable questions to ask to which it is virtually impossible to provide answers, because you just cannot do the requisite tests."

Finally, we have Dr. Mitchell A. Kline, a New York City dermatologist and melanoma expert affiliated with Cornell University Medical College and Weill NY-Presbyterian Medical Center. He is familiar with the effects cosmetics have on our bodies and says the cosmetics companies are, too. "It's exactly like cigarettes thirty years ago," he says. "We used to know that if you smoked, you got cancer. Now we know some of these ingredients are carcinogens."

Between these four experts, we have a lot of ground covered,

## ANIMAL TESTING

This book is not going to take on the moral debate of whether or not it is okay to test cosmetics ingredients on animals. That's not because we don't care about animals—in fact we've both been vegetarians or vegans to varying degrees of extremism because we very much *do* care. But the truth is, instead of testing on humans, scientists have used animals, and in order to understand how these chemicals work, we had to look at the animal data. "If you use something in large doses in a test animal over a short term, that approximates the use over long term in humans in much smaller doses," Schwarcz told us.

That said, not using toxic chemicals in the first place obviates the need for animal testing. So while we certainly appreciated the data when researching this book, almost all of the products we will recommend are light on "green chemistry" and heavy on pure, natural ingredients. And being cruelty-free is just one more compelling reason to go clean.

and a good balance. We imagine that some of the information you read will spark pretty strong feelings. You might think we're fear mongering or going a little soft, depending on where you fall on the zealot spectrum. You might also feel compelled to throw out everything in your bathroom (and maybe even throw out this book). Either way, our hope is that by the time you get to the end, you, too, will embrace our "why bother" motto. As in: why bother using that crap if I can't be sure that it's safe?

We'd also like to remind you of the second part to this maxim: why bother using that crap if the ingredients aren't even doing anything for your looks? In most cases, the problematic ones are not the important moisturizers or the age-fighting antioxidants—we're talking about preservatives, contaminants, dyes, foaming agents, things that make creams feel silky, and synthetic perfumes. What those do is improve the appearance of your product. They do not improve the appearance of your person, however. And some are making you look worse.

## CONTAMINANTS AND BYPRODUCTS

Because contaminants and byproducts are not intended ingredients, they won't turn up on labels. Contaminants include formaldehyde, nitrosamines, 1,4-dioxane, asbestos, lead, and mercury, to name only a few. These contaminants are very bad news, and while you won't always know from the label if they're in the bottle, they tend to be associated with certain ingredients that you can and should start avoiding. Cosmetics companies *can* guard against these contaminants through vacuum stripping, safe manufacturing, and other methods, and some do. Trouble is there's almost no way to know if the product you have your eye on has done this. Until companies are forced to list byproducts and contaminants on the label—at which point you'd better believe they'll be vacuum stripping their hearts out—take heed.

### 1,4-dioxane

This stealth compound, which has garnered much attention for its presence in baby products, is a byproduct of a process called ethoxylation and does not appear on labels.

**What it's used in:** According to a 2007 report by the Environmental Working Group, it's found in 22 percent of all personal care products[1]; a follow-up study by the EWG in 2009 found it in an alarming 67 percent of children's bath products.[2] It is also found in hair relaxers, dyes, shampoo, sunless tanners, body lotions, face creams, and anti-aging products.[3]

**How it's listed:** It may occur in products that list the ingredients PEG, polyethylene, polyethylene glycol, polyoxyethylene, as well as ingredients that end in "eth" or "oxynol." It may also be found in sodium laureth sulfate.

**Ugly factor:** Nothing about cancer is pretty.

**Risk factor:** Very high. It's a known carcinogen in animals and a probable one in humans, according to the Environmental Protection Agency (EPA), California's Prop 65 (which requires the state to provide a list of chemicals known to cause cancer or reproductive toxicity), and others.[4] Rats and mice that drank water contaminated with 1,4-D developed liver and nose cancers, while long-term studies of inhalation and skin contact showed that it affected the kidneys as well. It is readily absorbed through the skin, though once in the body it is broken down into other chemicals that we pee out (into our water).[5] While the FDA has not set guidelines for its use in cosmetics, it has set limits for its use in pills and spermicides at 10 parts per million (ppm)[6]; a 2007 study done by the Campaign for Safe Cosmetics found that many products exceeded that recommendation; some used as much as twice that amount.[7] Women also use an average of twelve products a day, so who knows how that math goes.

*Expert says:* "*1,4 really shows you how tricky byproducts can be. There seems to be a lot of concrete evidence on it that just makes you want to run in the other direction when you find out that it's not listed on labels.*" —Dr. Michael DiBartolomeis

## Aluminum Salts

These get a negative rap as the bad boy in antiperspirant. Aluminum is an abundant metal, traces of which can be found almost everywhere. Aluminum salts are used in antiperspirants to help seal the sweat gland and kill odor-causing bacteria.

*What it's used in:* Antiperspirant.

*How it's listed:* Aluminum chloride, aluminum chlorohydrate, aluminum hydroxybromide, and aluminum zirconium variations.

*Ugly factor:* Yellow stains on your wifebeaters; white stains on your little black dress.

*Risk factor:* Medium-high. Aluminum is a neurotoxin that has been linked to detrimental health effects in lab animals.[8] It was thought to be associated with Alzheimer's disease, but data is hotly debated. Some scientists suspect that the rise of antiperspirant use and the rise in breast cancer are related; others refute this claim.[9] One human study found it in breast tissue, which seems to indicate its ability to migrate from the armpit into the body.[10]

*One study says:* "*Aluminium is omnipresent in everyday life, and increased exposure is resulting in a burgeoning*

*body burden of this nonessential metal. Personal-care products are potential contributors to the body burden of aluminium, and recent evidence has linked breast cancer with aluminium-based antiperspirants.*"[11]

## Chemical Sunscreens

There are different ways to get protection from the sun. There are physical blockers such as zinc oxide and titanium dioxide, which literally block and deflect UVA and UVB rays, and then there are chemical sunscreens, which absorb UV rays before they can cause damage to the skin.

*What it's used in:* Sunscreens and most creams or makeup or lip balms with SPF.

*How it's listed:* There are many different kinds. They include padimate-O, PABA, benzophenone, oxybenzone, homosalate, octyl-methoxycinnamate, octinoxate. As a general rule, if the bottle boasts SPF and doesn't specify that it is a mineral or physical blocker, it contains some chemical sunscreen.

*Ugly factor:* Accidental aging by UVA rays, since many chemical sunscreens do not protect against them, and hormone disruption, which never plays well for skin.[12]

*Risk factor:* High. Padimate-O (aka PABA)—like titanium dioxide, a physical blocker—is a suspected carcinogen. (In most cases, titanium dioxide is off the hook because it is not absorbed by the skin unless it's in nanoparticle form—see

"Nanoparticles" on page 45.) Oxybenzone (benzophenone) has shown endocrine disruption in animals and is absorbed easily by skin—in fact, 97 percent of us have it in our urine.[13] Homosalate and octyl-methoxycinnamate (octinoxate) are also suspected of messing with hormones.[14]

*Expert says: "As far as protection goes, titanium dioxide is the best without a doubt. I think that the claims about oxybenzone are bogus, though. The amounts in there are trivial, and it doesn't get into the bloodstream in any meaningful way."* —Dr. Joseph Schwarcz

### Coal Tar

Made from bituminous coal, this stuff is used to treat patches of psoriasis and dandruff. It is also used to beat itches and is found in many of the synthetic colors in cosmetics.

*What it's used in:* Dandruff and psoriasis shampoo, anti-itch creams, cosmetics, hair dyes, and sometimes mouthwash and toothpaste.

*How it's listed:* When it's an active ingredient, such as in dandruff shampoo, the label will say coal tar or coal tar solution. Many dyes and synthetic colors are also made of coal tar, but because its constituent parts and not the whole are used, it won't say it on the label.

*Ugly factor:* It smells like a melting parking lot. Also, rashes.

*Risk factor:* High. Coal tar is a known human carcinogen according to a half dozen health and environmental agencies in the Western world.[15] In lab tests, it was shown to cause cancerous tumors when injected under the skin of animals. It's also an eye and skin irritant.[16] Several countries have it on their lists of banned or restricted ingredients.

*One study says:* *"The carcinogenicity of coal tar has been shown in animal studies and studies in occupational settings. . . . New, well-designed, epidemiological studies are necessary to assess the risk of skin tumors and other malignancies after dermatological use of coal tar."*[17]

### The "Ethanolamines": Diethanolamine (DEA), Triethanolamine (TEA), Monoethanolamine (MEA)/Ethanolamine (ETA)

In cosmetics, these can be emulsifiers, foaming agents, or used to adjust the pH levels of a product.[18] While DEA seems to be the most suspect of the bunch, both MEA and TEA also contain residual levels of DEA.

*What they're used in:* Lots of stuff such as facial cleansers, shampoos, body wash, hair colors, hair relaxers, and more.[19]

*How they're listed:* Too many ways to name, some of the most common ones being cocamide DEA, cocamide MEA, DEA-cetyl phosphate, DEA oleth-3 phosphate, lauramide DEA, linoleamide MEA, myristamide DEA, oleamide DEA, stearamide MEA, TEA lauryl sulfate, triethanolamine.

*Ugly factor:* A host of really nasty skin growths and conditions.[20]

*Risk factor:* High. The National Toxicology Program found a connection between topical application of DEA (and its related ingredients) and cancer in lab animals. The FDA expressed concern.[21] Amines can also combine in some cases to form nitrosamines, many of which are known carcinogens. The FDA's been worried about nitrosamine contamination in products since 1979.[22] DEA also appeared to screw with brain development in baby mice when applied topically to their pregnant mothers.[23]

*Expert says:* *"This is one of those cases where you have a clear situation of something being formed in most products—[nitrosamines]—and the longer it sits, the more likely you're going to have it in there."* —Dr. Michael DiBartolomeis

## Formaldehyde

This is what they use to embalm dead people. It shows up as an ingredient in cosmetics as a preservative, germicide, and is also released by other ingredients as a contaminant, so it's not always on the label.

*What it's used in:* Nail polish, antiperspirant, makeup, bubble bath, shampoo, baby lotions, "keratin" hair treatments, hair dye, and hair-growing products.

*How it's listed:* Cormalin; formic aldehyde; and variations, including methanal, methyl aldehyde, or oxymethane. It is also released (or "donated" as some scientists like to say) by DMDM hydantoin, quaternium-15, diazolidinyl urea, and imidazolidinyl urea—all very widely used ingredients in personal-care products.

**Ugly factor:** Rashes, pungent odor.

**Risk factor:** High. It is classified as carcinogenic to humans by the International Agency for Research on Cancer (IARC) and is associated with various kinds of cancer.[24] It can cause immune-system toxicity, liver problems, and can be an irritant and allergen. The CIR says it shouldn't be used in concentrations above 0.2 percent.[25] It is, though.[26] Chronic exposure is a big no-no.[27]

**Experts say:** *"Formaldehyde is in a lot of products, and it definitely could be of concern."* —Dr. Michael DiBartolomeis

*"DMDM Hydantoin converts to formaldehyde when it hits your skin, so we're basically pouring carcinogens onto our skin."* —Dr. Mitchell A. Kline

## Fragrance

Thanks to trade-secret laws, this can mean anything from natural essential oils (many of which are skin irritants) to synthetic cocktails containing as many as five hundred chemicals at a time (many of which are skin irritants, or worse). Fragrance can be inhaled, ingested, and absorbed through the skin.

**What it's used in:** Almost everything you use—perfume,

makeup, deodorant, hair dye, face wash, lotions, foot scrubs, cellulite cream, shampoo, conditioner—you name it.

**How it's listed:** Fragrance, perfume, parfum.

**Ugly factor:** Fragrance ingredients can cause unpleasant-looking dark or reddish patches, skin discoloration when exposed to sunlight, rashes and breakouts.

**Risk factor:** High, because of all the unknowns. Some fragrance ingredients are known neurotoxins; many are allergens or skin irritants; others exacerbate asthma.[28] There is also concern about synthetic musk's bioaccumulation, both in the tissue of the body and in the world. Fragrance also often disguises the presence of hormone-disrupting phthalates. (See "Phthalates.")

**Experts say:** *"I don't know if it would ever be possible to get trade secret laws changed—that's something lawyers would have to take on. I think it would be like trying to get Coca-Cola to reveal its formula."* —Dr. Dave Hobson

*"Do you know what I say when someone in a department store comes up to me and asks if they can spray me with perfume? I answer 'Sure, and do you mind if I pee on your leg?'"* —Dr. Joseph Schwarcz

### Hydroquinone (hydro-kwinn-oan)

Hydroquinone is an effective skin lightener. It is used in several prescription lotions as well as some over-the-counter ones and is popular in African and Asian markets (as well as among people trying to undo the visible effects of sun damage).[29] It can also be present as an impurity, which means it's not always on labels.

*What it's used in:* Skin lighteners, sunscreen, anti-aging creams, nail treatments.

*How it's listed:* Hydroquinone; variations of 1,4-benzene or di-hydroxybenzene; variations on hydroxyphenol.

*Ugly factor:* It can cause bluish-black lesions.

*Risk factor:* High. There is limited evidence of it causing cancer in lab animals. Ingesting the stuff can result in severe reactions in amounts as low as one gram, and death has occurred in a dose as low as five grams.[30] The CIR recommends that it be rinsed off after application, that it not be used in concentrations over 1 percent, and for limited periods of time only.[31] It is available at 2 percent OTC and 4 percent by prescription.[32] A few years ago the FDA proposed a ban on its use in OTC lotions. Industrial workers exposed to it suffered eye clouding.[33]

*Expert says: "This is one of those products that illustrates how people will go to dangerous lengths for a cosmetic result. And as a toxicologist, I don't want anyone to do that, but if someone can get their hands on it and doesn't follow the guidelines for usage, it can be very harmful."* —Dr. Dave Hobson

## Lead and Mercury

Both are metals that appear in cosmetics as contaminants, or as an ingredient called thimerosal, a mercury compound used as a preservative in mascara.[34]

**What it's used in:** Hard to say since they're usually contaminants, though we do know that the FDA, which conducted its own study in 2009, found lead in *all* of the lipsticks it tested. On average the levels exceeded the FDA's own guidelines for lead in candy by about ten times.[35] Lead acetate is in certain hair dyes, and thimerosal is used in mascara and other eye makeup.

**How they're listed:** Thimerosal and variations, but usually they're not listed.

**Ugly factor:** Things like depression and brain damage are never a good look.

**Risk factor:** Very high. Lead and mercury are both highly toxic to humans and can be absorbed through the skin and into the body.[36] If you don't die from poisoning, lead can still cause depression, aggressive behavior, miscarriages, and smaller babies. In children, evidence points to long-term learning disabilities.[37] Mercury is associated with renal failure, dementia, mental deterioration, and muscle tremors.[38]

**Experts say:** *"The more we know about lead, the more we realize that lower and lower and lower doses have an impact. Really you can make a pitch that if there's any level of any of these heavy metal products, they shouldn't be sold—there's just no rationale for it."* —Dr. Michael DiBartolomeis

*"If there is a detectable amount of lead in a cosmetic, I think*

*an effort should be made to have it removed from the formulation."* —Dr. Dave Hobson

## Nanoparticles

These are big news. Nanoparticles are used in cosmetics because they penetrate easily and may accumulate in body tissue. The use of nanoparticles in cosmetics and sunscreen is growing faster than in any other product categories, but their use across the board is through the roof.[39] They're very controversial.

*What it's used in:* Sunscreens, makeup, blush, acne treatments, anti-aging creams.[40] They're used in some mineral sunscreens to make whitish titanium dioxide look transparent.

*How it's listed:* In the United States and Canada, it's not. A new decree in the E.U., however, says that all future products must indicate clearly on the label if a given ingredient is used in nano form, and the company must also register a safety dossier with the European Commission.[41] If zinc oxide or titanium dioxide are listed, you want the particles to be larger than 100 nanometers. If it's not a brand you know and trust, you might have to call the company and ask them.

*Ugly factor:* Low.

*Risk factor:* Possibly quite high. Their smallness allows them to easily penetrate the skin and possibly cause cell damage. Ill effects include cancer, bioaccumulation in the body, and gene damage.[42]

*Expert says:* *"This is a complicated issue because some nanoparticles may have toxicity associated with them, while other ones might be okay. One thing is sure, though: any time you put a tiny nanosized particle into your body, it can get into places it shouldn't get into—like cells or DNA. I think in the future, we're going to be going back and saying, 'Why didn't we test these things better at the outset?'"* —Dr. Michael DiBartolomeis

## Parabens

You've probably heard of these puppies—they get a lot of media play. Parabens are preservatives used in every category of cosmetics, and are in 75 to 90 percent of all products on the market because they are a cheap and effective way to extend the shelf life of products.[43] Like phthalates, there are several different kinds.

*What it's used in:* Everything—makeup, shampoo, conditioner, lotions, scrubs. Everything.

*How it's listed:* Methyl/ethyl/butyl/isobutyl/propyl paraben, or variations including those prefixes and hydroxybenzoic acid or hydroxybenzoate or ester.

*Ugly factor:* One study showed that parabens can age the skin when exposed to UV light.[44]

*Risk factor:* Medium. It was previously thought that parabens did not penetrate the skin. We now know that they can migrate to body tissue.[45] Studies have shown that parabens mimic the hormone estrogen, which could affect both men and women. Parabens have also been found in breast tumor tissue (whether their estrogenic quality caused cancer cells to grow is unknown; more testing is needed).

*One study says:* *"The exposure issues are clear, and the exposed population is large, and these factors should provide the necessary impetus to investigate this potential issue of public health."*[46]

## Petroleum Distillates/Solvents

Extracted by distillation during the refining of crude oil, these are usually some kind of clear liquid used to dissolve other substances.[47] Petroleum distillates/solvents should not be confused with petrolatum, which is the stuff in Vaseline or its cousin paraffin. While all of these substances are indeed related—be it jelly, wax, oil, or solvent—physiochemical differences account for the solvents' higher toxicity.[48] But even if some are harmless, given from where they're sourced, we generally avoid the whole petrochemical family.

*What it's used in:* It's especially common in mascara as well as other makeup, hair, nail, and skin care products.

*How it's listed:* Petroleum distillate, stoddard solvent, light liquid paraffin.

*Ugly factor:* Low.

*Risk factor:* Medium-high. In an occupational study of people exposed to petroleum distillate solvents, it was concluded that they increased the risk of developing undifferentiated connective tissue disease (UTCD).[49] The symptoms of UTCD range from rashes to an enlarged heart, with a lot in between.[50] According to the EPA, aspirations of small amounts can be dangerous.[51] They are also sometimes contaminated with butadiene, which is a carcinogen, and the E.U. has banned certain petroleum distillates in cosmetics.[52]

*EPA report says:* *"Aspiration of small amounts of these chemicals into the lung can cause chemical pneumonia, pulmonary damage, and death."*[53]

## p-Phenylenediamine (fen-a-leen-die-a-meen)

Found in most hair dyes, including some hennas, p-Phenylenediamine (p-PD) has been used to dye things since 1890.[54] It is a hot-button ingredient that has had the FDA and other health agencies on watch for a long time, though efforts to restrict or ban its—and other hair dye ingredients'—use have been defeated over and over. There is also concern about how it interacts with other chemicals in hair dyes.

*What it's used in:* Hair dye, hair bleach, colored shampoo, henna dyes.

*How it's listed:* 1,4-Benzenediamine, p-Phenylenediamine, 4-Phenylenediamine.

***Ugly factor:*** Eczema, rashes.

***Risk factor:*** Medium-high. Exposure can cause bronchial problems, nervous system damage, severe allergic reactions, and in some studies it was linked to bladder cancer (though that is hotly debated). There is also evidence of it being a neurotoxin.[55]

***One study says:*** *"These results suggest that p-Phenylenediamine can induce DNA damage and accumulation of [certain] mutant proteins; this may be one of the possible mechanisms that cause genotoxic carcinogenesis in the urothelial cells* [i.e., can cause bladder cancer]"[56]

## Phenoxyethanol (fen-oxy-etha-nol)

An organic chemical compound, phenoxyethanol has been touted as a friendly preservative-alternative to parabens. This has made it especially popular with natural and fake-natural companies.

***What it's used in:*** Since it's a preservative, it's used across the board. It is popular in face lotions and cleansers. It is also used in some fragrance, in which case it won't be on the label.

***How it's listed:*** Phenoxyethanol, variations including 2-phenoxy and ethanol, 2-hydroxyethyl phenyl ether, etc.

***Ugly factor:*** Some studies have shown it to be a skin and eye irritant.[57]

*Risk factor:* Medium. Phenoxyethanol has been shown to produce significant reproductive and developmental toxicity.[58] While the opposite has also been reported, its use in cosmetics is restricted (but not banned) in Japan and Europe.[59] Even the FDA issued a warning about the presence of phenoxyethanol in a nipple cream, saying to keep the babies away from it.[60]

*The FDA warning says: "Phenoxyenthanol, a preservative that is primarily used in cosmetics and medications, can also depress the central nervous system and may cause vomiting and diarrhea, which can lead to dehydration in infants."*[61]

## Phthalates (thall-ates)

Pronounce it however you want, but these are important to get to know. (We say *"thall-ates,"* but we still get corrected all the time.) This is a group of chemical compounds used in plastics, water bottles, cosmetics, perfume, pesticides, toys—you name it. They're everywhere.[62]

*What it's used in:* Perfume, most fragrances in most products, nail polish, nail strengtheners, eyelash glue, hair spray, lotion.

*How it's listed:* In fragrance it's not listed at all. Elsewhere, anything that has "phthalate" in its name. Also listed as DBP, DEHP, DMP, DEP, with variations on dibutyl/diethyl ester, or variations on 1,2-benzenedicarboxylate.

*Ugly factor:* High, if you consider hormonal acne, obesity, and reproductive defects to be unappealing.

*Risk factor:* Very high. Phthalates are known hormone disruptors, suspected carcinogens, are possibly toxic to fetuses, and can cause birth defects in male babies.[63] They can also impair fertility and are a suspected cause of endometriosis and polycystic ovarian syndrome (PCOS).[64] They do not accumulate in the body but because they are so commonly used, women have very high levels of exposure—that little adds up to a lot.

*One study says:* *"DBP* [dibutylphthalate] *is an environmentally dangerous hormone that disrupts the pathways of testicular differentiation\* in genetically male animals."*[65]


## Propylene Glycol (PG), Ethylene Glycol, Diethylene Glycol, Polyethylene Glycol (PEG)

Propylene glycol can be derived naturally, but it usually is not. It is widely used in small amounts as a moisture-sealer and as a penetration enhancer (which helps carry things into the skin). It is nontoxic when ingested and easily biodegrades.[66] Ethylene is often used to make products "gentler." Polyethylene glycol is widely used in so-called natural cosmetics under other names.

*What it's used in:* Lots of things—shampoo, makeup, baby washes, lotions, foundation, soaps.

*How it's listed:* Often just by the names listed above or 1-2 propanediol. Polyethylene glycol (PEG) and polypropylene

---

\*In this study done on frogs, 17 percent of the tadpoles developed something akin to ovaries when they should have developed testicles.

glycol (PPG) are related. You will also see variations on 1,2-dihydroxypropane and variations on methylethylene glycol.

**Ugly factor:** Rashes, acne.

**Risk factor:** Medium. In the family of glycols used in cosmetics, PG is considered the most safe, though it penetrates skin easily and in high enough doses can have ill effects.[67] PEG was known to cause systemic toxicity in patients who applied it to damaged skin.[68] Some experts say the biggest risk involved is impurities. PEG contaminants can include the carcinogens 1,4-dioxane, lead, nickel, and arsenic.

**One study says:** *"PEGs are readily absorbed through damaged skin and are associated with contact dermatitis and systemic toxicity in burn patients. PEGs were not sensitizing to normal skin."*[69]

## Sodium Laureth Sulfate and Sodium Lauryl Sulfate

SLES and SLS are surfactants widely used in shampoo and other things that foam and clean. They're among the most commonly used because they are effective at cutting through oil, and they're inexpensive. Some companies have begun phasing them out and even now advertise their absence.

**What it's used in:** Shampoo, soap, body wash, toothpaste, bubble bath, face wash, mascara, conditioner, baby washes, exfoliants.

*How it's listed:* Sodium lauryl/laureth sulfate, sodium dodecyl sulfate, sodium salt sulphuric acid, monododecyl ester, other variations including sodium sulfate or sodium salt combined with other chemicals, and PEG lauryl sulfate and variations.

*Ugly factor:* Rashes, scalp scabs, canker sores, and stripped color and shine from hair.[70]

*Risk factor:* High. SLES and SLS penetrate the skin and scalp easily and cannot be metabolized by the liver. They are possibly endocrine disruptors, and common skin, scalp and eye irritants. But the biggest concern is contamination with 1,4-dioxane.[71] (See "1,4-dioxane.")

*Expert says: "Not everything we put on our skin goes into our body. It depends on how big the particles are. So certain substances are not absorbed into the body, while other substances such as SLS are known to be absorbed into body tissues, and that is frightening."* —Dr. Mitchell A. Kline

## Talc

Talc is a mineral used in its loose form as talcum powder, the main ingredient in baby powder. For decades there has been concern (and confusion) around talcum powder and its link to asbestos, due in part to contamination fears as well as to its similar chemical composition. Most talc now is asbestos-free.

*What it's used in:* Baby powder, liquid powder, eye shadows, face powders, sunscreens.

***How it's listed:*** Talc, talcum powder.

***Ugly factor:*** Low.

***Risk factor:*** Medium. Several studies have linked talc exposure to ovarian cancer. In some cases frequent application of talcum powder to the genital area appeared to significantly elevate risk.[72] Other studies have found no causal connection.[73] The data is inconclusive but some doctors advise against its use (and we do, too). Inhalation studies in some animals have also shown talc to be a possible lung irritant and carcinogen—which is not cute for baby.[74]

***One study says:*** *"These results suggest that women with certain genetic variants may have a higher risk of ovarian cancer associated with genital talc use. Additional research is needed on these interactions and the underlying biological mechanisms."*[75]

## Toluene (toll-you-een)

This is a stinky solvent used in a number of things, including paint thinners and in the production of cola syrup.[76] It is also used in high concentrations in many nail products. (Not to be confused with butylated hydroxy*toluene* (BHT), which is a different but also unfavorable ingredient that we will cover in a later chapter.)

***What it's used in:*** Nail polish, nail hardener, a 1991 study done by the EPA found it in fragrance formulations, and in 2006

IFRA deemed it unsafe so it recommends that "toluene has to be kept as low as practicable."[77] Comforting?

*How it's listed:* Toluene; toluol; variations on methylbenzene and phenylmethane; of course, in the case of fragrance it will not be listed.

*Ugly factor:* Brittle nails.

*Risk factor:* High. Benzene, which is derived from toluene, is a bone marrow poison related in some studies to leukemia, and it is a toxin that can make you high or nauseous/lightheaded/ill from inhaling it (huffers, take note).[78] Toluene is also believed to increase the risk of spontaneous abortion: women with occupational exposure had four times as many miscarriages as their unexposed counterparts (see study quote below).[79] It enters the body through inhalation and skin contact and does not exit easily via the normal channels.

*One study says: "Specific exposure to toluene seems to be associated with a risk of foetal loss."*[80]

## Triclosan

Triclosan is a synthetic antimicrobial agent that also has antibacterial, antifungal, and antiviral properties. In other words it's a very powerful germ killer, and it's used in a wide variety of products.[81]

*What it's used in:* Almost everything from soaps to toothpaste, to acne treatments, antiperspirants, and lipstick.

***How it's listed:*** As triclosan and a dizzying and confusingly long list of other ways that involve chloro and dichlorophenoxy. (For a complete list, see Skin Deep's online database at www.cosmeticsdatabase.com).

***Ugly factor:*** It's a known skin irritant.

***Risk factor:*** Medium. While it's considered relevant for use in the antimicrobial soaps in hospitals[82]—where people are at high-risk for contracting certain infections—there's no data supporting that everyday use has any health benefits.[83] To the contrary, there is concern that regular exposure could cause resistant strains of bacteria to form (similar to what happens when antibiotics are overused).[84] It also stays in our bodies and in our water. It was found in human breast milk and plasma, and in more than one animal study it has impacted thyroid function.[85]

***One study says:*** *"Exposure to low levels of triclosan disrupts thyroid hormone-associated gene expression and can alter the rate of thyroid hormone-mediated postembryonic anuran development."*[86]

## THE LABEL GAME

Before 1973, cosmetics manufacturers were not required to list their ingredients; it was only with the introduction of the Fair Packaging and Labeling Act that companies finally had to reveal what the hell was in their products. Here's a summary of the most important things to know.[87]

1. Ingredients are listed in descending order of concentration. So if the first ingredient in that $150 anti-wrinkle cream is water, it means you're probably being ripped off. Because companies are required to use the chemical nomenclature—and because most of us don't speak chemistry—ingredient lists can get pretty confusing. Our list and online resources should help, though.

2. Any ingredient used in a concentration lower than 1 percent can be listed in any order the manufacturer chooses, and there is no way to tell where the higher-concentrated ingredients end and the 1-percenters begin.[88]

3. Certain words used on labels and in ads are unregulated. This includes the promises to make you younger, smoother, and hotter, as well as the use of phrases like "dermatologist-tested," "allergy-tested," "hypoallergenic," "non-irritating," "gentle," "herbal," "botanical," "natural," and "cruelty-free."[89] Get it through your pretty heads: for now, *the only legitimate information on the bottle or box is the ingredients list, and the order in which they are listed.*

4. Actually, not so fast. Certain products are classified as both drugs and cosmetics, and in those cases, the "active" is listed first. Drugs in cosmetics—like the aluminum in antiperspirant or the avobenzone in sunscreen—are subject to pre-market approval. This labeling can be misleading, since the logical assumption would be that the active ingredient is also the main ingredient. Not so.

5. Trade-secret laws protect companies from having to disclose the hundreds of ingredients used to make the "fragrance" or "parfum" in your products, which means they're not on the label. At all. Reread the sections on

fragrance and phthalates for a reminder as to why that's bad news.

So there you have it. Ingredient lists do not on their own clear up confusion, but they are the most honest thing about the products we buy. But even if you're reading labels, how do you know what that nine-syllable word even means? You should read (and reread, and reread) our ingredients-to-avoid list, obviously, but beyond that you have two options.

### The Deep-Dive Way to Learn

This is the option that requires you to really learn how to read labels. We recommend you do this, but we also know it's not for everyone. If you do want to, start with the Skin Deep: Cosmetic Safety Database—an invaluable (and overwhelming) resource; we talk about it on pages 59–60. Then there's good old Google, where you can investigate every listed ingredient and attempt to separate the facts from the fiction. We've spent hundreds of hours doing this. It has its benefits and pitfalls. Besides the fact that it can get spooky, it's also unreliable: there are data gaps and biases that taint both sides of the argument.

Finally, there are also books like Ruth Winter's indispensable *A Consumer's Dictionary of Cosmetic Ingredients*. She takes a middle-of-the-road approach, and is a reliable source of information on pretty much any ingredient in cosmetics. You can find other books we recommend in our resources section at the end of this book.

## The Wading Pool Way To Learn

This is the easier option. If you don't want to become an ingredient whiz, here are some rules of thumb:

1. Products with ingredients you can pronounce are more likely to be nice to you in the morning.
2. Toxicologists and supermodels alike will tell you that the fewer ingredients there are, the better.
3. Finally, take the time to get to know companies' ingredient policies, and pick a few you can trust. There are some truly amazing and transparent companies out there. They want to answer your questions, they list ingredients in a font size and color you can read, and they make clean products. Once you know who they are, you can sit back a little and buy with ease. Some stores, too, are doing the hard work for you. Whole Foods carries some things we love, and so do luxurious websites like Spirit Beauty Lounge, the Nature of Beauty, and others. Again, see our resource section for places you can shop without having to think about it too much.

---

### HOW TO USE THE
### SKIN DEEP COSMETIC SAFETY DATABASE

Cosmeticsdatabase.com is a beast, and we mean that in the best possible way. Created by the Environmental Working Group's Campaign for Safe Cosmetics, it is an exhaustive online tool with tens of thousands of product listings, including complete ingredient lists and cross-referenced data information about those ingredients. You can search by brand, product, or ingredient and then sift through a thorough summary of the data that exists about it. Of course, the fact that it's a database means it has some glitches.

"Skin Deep can be overwhelming, there is no doubt," says the campaign's co-founder Stacy Malkan. "It is an amazing tool and a huge step forward. It was the first time we really had a window into the whole landscape of what is used in products and how toxic they are. It's taken us really far, but it's one step, one tool for consumers to look into the products they're using."

So you shouldn't just type in a product name then freak out based solely on the one-to-ten safety rating that pops up at the top of the screen. As one example: if you look up Dr. Hauschka mascara, they do have a high rating because "fragrance" is listed on the labels. Because that word can mean almost anything, it gets an eight—which sort of skews the safety rating of any product that lists it. But having looked into Dr. Hauschka, we trust that its "fragrance" is all-natural, so in our minds, it gets a pass. Malkan agrees. "I would trust Dr. Hauschka because I know that company, have been to their headquarters, and know they have strong philosophies. So that's one where you might question a ranking in Skin Deep or call the company to ask them what they are using in their fragrance."

If you're not the kind of person who wants to bother with writing a company to ask them what they use, your best bet is doing some reading (like this book, say) and figure out which brands you trust and which ones you don't.

## "NATURAL," "ORGANIC," "BOTANICAL," AND OTHER BULLSHIT CLAIMS

These days, there are so many "green" and "natural" claims and just as many certification labels popping up on bottles that there's even an anti-greenwasher website devoted to what these little icons do and do not mean. Guess how many it reviews? Two hundred ninety-nine. That should give you an idea of how bogus most of these "green" labels are.

In the United States, in addition to having no government agency overseeing this stuff, there is no nongovernmental certifier for cosmetics that you can wholly trust, either. As a result, some companies have begun using food-grade organics in order to earn the USDA Organic seal. As we were finishing this book, the National Organic Standard Board (NOSB) was proposing that the use of the *word* organic on labels be regulated. (The PCPC opposed it, though, and we're betting it has more money than the NOSB, so we are not holding our breath.) Meanwhile, some legitimate organic companies were suing others for alleged misuse of the word. Clearly, there is confusion all around, but for now, know that the USDA Organic seal means something, while the word "organic" most likely does not.

So, ditch your body cream and read the next chapter. With that you'll be 70 percent chem-free in no time and excited to try the wonders of truly clean products on your face.

---

## DON'T-PANIC TIPS
## ON PURGING YOUR PRODUCTS

At this point, one of two things may be happening. Either you're ready to storm your bathroom with a giant garbage bag in tow, or you're thinking it's time to put this book down and unlearn the last twenty pages. If it's the latter, try not to panic. We both felt the same when we started reading about chemicals, but it's less overwhelming than you think. Here are a few tips of attack based on what we did.

1. Ignore your face for now. It's a smaller surface area, which means less of any given product is likely to make its way in. Also, these are the products you are most attached to—makeup, wrinkle cream, face wash—so when you're good and ready, (i.e., after you've read the face and makeup chapters), you can begin to tackle them.

2. Take a look at the products you use on your whole body, especially any moisturizer you slather on regularly. Change that out first. If you want to skip ahead to the "The Body Guide" on page 181—by all means. Know that there are plenty of clean, affordable options to swap it with. Your body wash or soap can go next—that's also an easy switch-out.

3. We're going to start you off with hair in the next chapter, and there's a reason for that. Even the most finicky girl among us has experimented with her hair. A cut, a color, some new product her hairdresser sold her on—our hair is transformative, fun to play with, and less delicate than our skin. It's where we both started and quickly found great products and learned new techniques to keep ours healthy. Now it's your turn.

# 4

# Your Hair

Hopefully at this point you're a little pissed and primed to start cleaning up your act. Off the bat, let's get one thing clear: plastic surgery notwithstanding, there's not a whole lot you can do about most of your features. It just depends which line you were in when they were giving out genes. The goal, of course, is to be at peace with what you can't control (easier said than done) and focus instead on those things you can, like your hair. Hair defines your look, makes a statement about who you are, and reflects your health all at once. Best of all, it's comparatively easy to get it to look how you want— unless you're trying to make it look completely and permanently different from what nature intended.

To better understand what your hair is and how it works—not to mention how your current products are screwing it up—read on. We'll tell you how your scalp and hair function, what ingredients are typically used in your products, and why you should avoid them. Then— the fun part—we'll recommend products and at-home recipes we particularly love. You will also hear about Siobhan's attempt to detox her highlights, and Alexandra's adventure in not washing her hair at all.

## MEET YOUR SCALP

Your scalp is one of the most absorbent parts of your body—more than the face where you slather anti-aging cream, or the legs you douse post-shave. The scalp is basically a sponge that sops up whatever you put on it. It's also your most sensitive skin, and it extends all the way down to your eyes, so it stands to reason we should be extra careful what goes on or near it. And yet, for most women—and definitely for us—there's a disconnect between our hair and our health. After all, you would never spritz your arms with something that smelled and stung like hair spray, or massage the burny chemicals of hair relaxers into your thighs.

That's the same disconnect that sent us down the rabbit hole in the first place. As you'll recall, it was an expensive formalde-hyde-laced hair treatment that first woke us up to the scary realities of the chemicals in our beauty products. And because we wrote this book to save you the trouble of finding out the hard way how bad this stuff is for you, here's a primer on why you should be extra careful with your head.

Your scalp is made up of five layers, the first of which is home to around one hundred thousand hair follicles (more, for some reason, if you're blonde).[1] The follicle produces hair by packing dead cells together that are made mostly of a protein called ker-atin. At the base of each follicle are sebaceous glands. These get a bad rap because sebaceous is a disgusting word, and sebum—that oily lubricant it forms—is the oft-cited culprit of greasy skin and acne. But sebum plays an important role in the appear-ance and health of hair, making it shine and bounce. It even pro-tects the scalp against infection.

Correction: when it's there, sebum protects against infection.

Chances are good that if you're using conventional hair products, you're stripping that helpful sebum and preventing it from working its magic, which in turn makes your scalp more exposed to the chemicals you're putting on it. That means that some of what you rub into it (shampoo), let sit on it (conditioner), leave on it (defrizzer), and color it with (high-tox dyes, anyone?) is going straight into your scalp.

So what happens while the chemicals from your hair products are still in your body, hanging out in your blood, and making pit stops in your organs? That depends on the chemical. Some ingredients will be peed out later, but not all chemicals leave your body quite so quickly. Some are even known to hang out for the better part of a year. And since many of us have spent a whole life with handfuls of gunk in our hair, chemical-relaxing it into submission, or coloring it so religiously that we've forgotten our natural hue, it's fair to say almost all of us have some cleaning up to do.

## Shampoo

Shampoo, named for a still-popular Indian head massage (*chāmpo* in Hindi), didn't become the product we know and love until the 1930s. While the Indians used oils, the main ingredients in our shampoos today are detergents, water, surfactants, and alcohol.[2] Surfactants are wetting agents that help trap oil and the dirt stuck to it, allowing the water to rinse it all off. Unfortunately, in the process, this also strips hair of its natural oils. This makes our hair feel oh-so clean (which we love), but it also perpetuates a cycle that demands more and more products.

The surfactants used in most shampoos—usually sodium laureth sulfate (SLES) or its sister sodium lauryl sulfate (SLS)—can cause unsightly rashes on many of us. Even worse, however, is when SLES is ethoxylated—a cheap process meant to soften the harshness of the chemical—it produces a carcinogen called 1,4-dioxane.[3] Consult Chapter 3 for a reminder, but the kicker is that 1,4-D doesn't even get listed on labels because it's not what the FDA likes to call an "intended ingredient." That means it's a byproduct. To which we say: "But it's a known byproduct, and it's an avoidable byproduct, and it causes cancer, so shouldn't that mean it goes on the label or—crazy talk—gets banned?" But we digress.

Like sulfates, the other potentially dangerous ingredients in your shampoo aren't active ones: it's the preservatives, the fragrance, and the additives you need to worry about. Popular ones in shampoo are foam boosters such as lauramide DEA or cocamide DEA and MEA, and the preservatives DMDM hydantoin and methylparaben. DEA is fine on its own, but when it sits on the shelf (which is to say always), it can react with the other chemicals to form nitrosamines[4]—potent and easily absorbed carcinogens linked to stomach, esophagus, liver, and bladder cancer.[5] Meanwhile, some preservatives, such as DMDM, release "small" amounts of formaldehyde; parabens might eff up thyroid and estrogen levels; and phthalates are known hormone disruptors that might also interfere with neurological functions. This stuff is in almost all—if not all-all—the shampoos we've ever used, even the ones for babies.

When you switch to a clean shampoo, you will probably notice a few things. First, it won't lather like Pantene. You will be tempted, then, to pour more into your palm, thinking you just aren't using enough to get a good suds. Don't do this.

## WASH YOUR HAIR BACKWARD

We sat down with natural hair care legend Horst Rechelbacher, who founded Aveda in 1978, and he got us to drink sparkling water spritzed with hair products from his Intelligent Nutrients line— because, yes, it is *that* clean. He also told us that if we wanted to feel "clean like a whistle" in the shower, we'd have to start doing things backward.

"When you wash your hair, try using your conditioner first," he said flatly. "If you want to go all the way, put oils on your scalp, give yourself a nice massage, and then comb it through. Next, wet it down, put conditioner all over your hair and then also all over your body. Wash yourself with the conditioner, then rinse it all off. Then, you use shampoo. Rinse it off, and you won't need conditioner again. If your hair is tangly, put a little oil on your hands, and then comb it through." That's it, he says. "You will feel very pure."

It's as counterintuitive as it gets, but if you aren't using harsh soaps on your hair, it makes a lot of sense. Your hair and scalp will lap up the beneficial (and, compared to shampoo, expensive) oils, and the light wash at the end just rinses the excess. That means no oily residue left on your skin, but plenty sopped up into your locks. Win-win.

They don't lather the same way because they don't contain foam boosters and harsh detergents. Use only a quarter-size amount, rub your hands together, then run your hands over your scalp and then to the hair ends. If you aren't using silicone- and plastic-based leave-ins, your hair simply won't need the kind of harsh washing you're accustomed to. But rest assured: your hair *is* getting clean.

You will probably notice immediate changes. Your hair will feel smoother, look shinier, and that stubborn scalp itch or rash you've had forever? It'll be gone in a week. Siobhan had the worst rash where her hairline meets the back of her neck. It had been variously diagnosed by dermatologists as psoriasis, seborrheic dermatitis, eczema, and plain old dandruff, so she's tried more prescription topicals than she can count—but nothing worked. Then she changed her shampoo, and guess what happened?

---

## THE POCAHONTAS THEORY
### Why Alexandra Stopped Washing Her Hair

Every woman has had at least one hairdresser advise her to wash her mane less frequently. That's because even those who aren't on team clean recognize that our shampoos are harsher than they need to be, and our daily washing is excessive. But what about just not washing *at all*?

Here's the disclaimer: I happen to be the ideal candidate for dirty hair. My mass of curls has always been a bit more Brillo pad than Botticelli. And while I didn't always love it (or even *like* it—kids can be mean), I've learned to appreciate it in my adult life. Among its more endearing qualities: it never gets too greasy. I was already down to bi-weekly washings (as instructed by hairdressers), so when I started reading online testimonials from curlies and straights who have embraced what is called the "no poo" movement—as in, lame for no shampoo—I was intrigued.

Not washing my hair made immediate sense to me, especially since shampoo entered our lives only seventy years ago. What did Pocahontas do? Probably not foam her lovely locks in Herbal Essences. The dirty theory, then, posits that if you stop washing and conditioning your hair altogether, eventually you will restore your scalp's natural balance, producing the perfect amount of sebum for healthy, beautiful hair—sans grease.

Given how clever our bodies are, it's not such a leap, though I realize it takes a certain degree of unlearning to embrace this logic. Consider, however, that conditioner was popularized because shampoo was making hair look like crap. Likewise, over time, the dull build-up created by conditioner sent us right back into the abusive arms of shampoo. May I remind you that hair care in the United States is a multibillion dollar industry?

So I tried it. I had recently left a job and was freelancing from home, minimizing witnesses. And actually, my biggest fear wasn't not shampooing, but not conditioning. How was I going to get the comb through my hair in the shower? I used to leave in a handful of the thickest (and most toxic) variety daily. Nonetheless, I went cold turkey.

And . . . drum roll please . . . not much happened! Amazingly, my hair looked pretty close to how I tried to make it look *with* product. It never got itchy or nasty (which did happen when I was using chemy conditioner and didn't wash it for a few days), and it became oddly more responsive to styling. If I wanted it straighter, a quick flat iron would do the trick. Extra volume? Some finger plying at my scalp sufficed. Combing it was easy, maybe even easier, than with conditioner. Huh.

That's not to say there weren't pitfalls. While the top half was softer than ever, the ends were especially coarse—a glitch that conditioner used to help mask. There is a technique whereby you run a washcloth down your hair when it's wet and that moves the oils along the hair shaft, eventually bringing life to your dry ends. It works, but it was a bit tedious for me. There was also the smell. It's not that it stank; even after smoky party nights it was surprisingly self-cleaning. But it smelled like hair, and I wanted it to smell like girl hair.

While it's probably not for everyone, experimenting with the dirty is still a solid idea, if only to give your mop a break from the excess of product—there's a financial incentive there, too. If yours is not too long, you may see the benefits rather quickly. But remember, since your hair is caught in the punishing cycle of harsh shampoos that strip everything out, it may get greasy at first. That's where the baking soda–vinegar "wash" from "The Hair Guide" really comes in handy, on page 82.

I still don't wash my hair—for a year and counting. But I have tinkered to find the best technique. I now use clean conditioners, especially on my ends, as well as Intelligent Nutrients' hair treatment, which leaves a delightful smell post-rinse. I've had a few trims, and the natural oils have definitely migrated down my hair shaft without too much coaxing, and my hair looks healthier for it. While I'm clearly not the pure no-product devotee like some of those no-pooers, dirty has started to feel like the new clean.

---

## Conditioner

Conditioner predates shampoo, if you consider that people have used natural oils for centuries to make their hair silky. It only really got its commercial wings after the creation of shampoo—because when you remove all of your natural oils, you need to replace them, or your hair will look like garbage. In addition to harsh cleansing and treatments, the sun, dyeing, poor diet, and even aging can affect how dry your hair is. Thankfully, science has taken conditioner to new heights: coating, glossing, shining, detangling, and volumizing like never before. Different chemical compounds play different roles in this, and not all of them are bad for you.

Most conditioners include humectants, artificial fragrance, preservatives, and finishing ingredients like silicones. Silicones coat the hair to make it more manageable and slick, but they're nonbiodegradable and completely synthetic. Also, no matter how much vitamin E or protein the label promises is in the bottle, it won't make a difference to your hair. The hair is dead, and no amount of goo is going to bring it back to life. If you're intent on having the shiniest, most manageable, and healthy hair on the block, you need to take care of yourself with omega-3s and vitamins, stay out of the sun, use the low setting on your hair dryer, and get one of the amazing conditioners we recommend at the end of the chapter.

That's not to say conditioner doesn't serve its purpose. Its basic role is to make your hair look pretty by maintaining a pH between 2.5 and 3.5. Hair has a kind of scaly surface that tightens up when it comes into contact with an acidic environment—like conditioner, giving it a smoother appearance.[6] That explains why hippies, for example, advocate using apple cider vinegar to make your hair soft and shiny. It has a pH around 3, which is why it works like a charm. This is all very encouraging news: conditioner is one of the easiest products to replace because its function is simple and effective, and the market for alternatives is well-populated with standouts for all budgets.

Conditioner, even the rinse-off kind, is formulated to coat the hair. So the chemicals in your conditioner stay with you all day and all night, getting into your body through your scalp, rubbing on your skin, getting on your clothes, sleeping with you on your pillow (hello, zits!). Obviously, this goes for any product that is left in your hair. Which brings us to . . .

## Leave-In Hair Products: Hair Spray, Hair Gel, Defrizzers, and More

Like conditioner, styling products are formulated specifically to stay with you. But unlike conditioner, we don't even pretend to rinse these out, even though they can leak into our skin on contact and can be inhaled on application. It's creepy, especially when you consider that some of their ingredients are capable of making you sick, itchy, and rashy. And it's annoying when you consider that some of their ingredients are capable of making your hair ugly, limp, and dry.

Take **hair spray**. No one thinks hair spray is natural, per se, but most women don't realize it may be as bad for you as those aerosol cans are for the ozone layer. A brief trip down hair spray–history lane offers a cautionary tale.

One ingredient in the hair spray our moms used is vinyl chloride monomer (VCM). Popularized in the late 1950s as an alternative to chlorofluorocarbons (CFCs), it was the *de rigueur* propellant in hair spray until 1974. Amazing stuff, everyone thought, until VCM was exposed as a toxic carcinogen that caused cancer in lab animals and humans, not to mention being potentially fatal if inhaled.[7] It's also flammable. Let's lay some general ground rules here, ladies: any beauty product that warns of high flammability should probably not come into contact with that beautiful mug of yours.

Now, we'll give you an idea of how ethical the beauty industry can be: even after makers of VCM—as well as beauty companies using it in their hair sprays—learned definitively in 1971 that it could cause tumors in humans, they were not quick to act. It wasn't until 1974 that the manufacturers took action, and even then they didn't cease production or sales of it; they merely upped the price to discourage its use.[8] These were clearly people with your health in mind.

Logic would say that once the cat was out of the bag, this nasty chem would be replaced with a safe one, and that while cosmetics companies were reformulating, they might as well reformulate to exclude other chemicals known to be problematic. But as recently as November 2008, a report showed that pregnant women exposed to hair spray at work doubled their chances of giving birth to a son with birth defects. The suspected culprit? Yet another kind of chemical—none other than your friendly neighborhood phthalates.[9] A 2009 report by the National Endocrine Society made the most definitive statement to date about phthalates' role as endocrine disruptors—affirming what other studies, experts, and government groups have been saying for decades. And yet these are probably in just about every leave-in styling product you've ever heard of, and when it's in the fragrance, it doesn't even get listed on the label.

Then there's **hair gel**, a favorite among curly and short-haired girls. Aside from drying out your hair with alcohol, and making it gross to the touch, it manages to combine a host of the worst chemicals we've encountered. You know, the ones that enable or increase penetration of chemicals, release formaldehyde, and are contaminated with carcinogens. We say skip it: there are natural alternatives like aloe and good options from lines like Intelligent Nutrients.

**Curl creams** are another popular category for this set. But despite their thick consistency, these often contain very drying ingredients such as alcohol (the last thing curls need), fragrance, formaldehyde releasers such as DMDM hydantoin, 1,4-dioxane-contaminated PEGs, along with propylene glycol, parabens, and other junk that sits on (or seeps into) your scalp all day. If you're super attached to your formula, we recommend you save it for a rainy day (literally) and find another one you can use regularly. Start by getting a gentler shampoo and opting for nondrying, nontoxic leave-ins—we promise you'll be glad you did. It took Alexandra months to persuade her ringletted sister to switch to a nontox routine. We're pleased to report that said sister now loves her hair more than ever. (An added benefit: once the chemical products disappeared from her regimen, so did the "mystery" scalp and neck bumps that had been cropping up for years.)

We're not sure that anyone under age seventy uses **pomade**, so we'll skip that one—it's mostly waxes and oils—and get to **defrizzers**. There are two main kinds: those made with an aloe-alcohol-water mix, and those that rely on silicones that coat the shaft. The former can be fine; just check ingredient labels to be sure they're clear of parabens and fragrance. But in our opinion, silicones are dangerous no matter how sleek they make your hair. They also build up on the hair shaft, cause breakouts on your face and back, and they're synthetic. As alternatives, we're partial to argan oil smoothed over dry hair, and pure aloe on wet hair.

"We don't use plasticizers," says Rechelbacher, who sold Aveda to Estée Lauder in 1997 and recently launched his own Intelligent Nutrients—a USDA Organic skin, hair, and body line that is also certified by the Soil Association. "They [companies] all do, because it's stiff, and it holds. Then, they mix them with silicones to make it silky. And then you have a real problem. Silicones are nonrecyclable. They do not break down—it's not possible. How scary is that?" he says. "Silicone can break down only so far as microdust, where it becomes what it was: sand. But worse, it's combined with petrochemicals with huge, gigantic machinery, [then it's] bound together, and it is no longer possible to take them apart. That is scary. If you inhale those, they're with you. That's it." Hold on, it gets worse: "I think one of the most dangerous things you can do is combine silicones with petrochemicals in beauty products."

So skip silicones altogether. You can find them on your labels usually containing "ethicone" such as dimethicone, trimethicone, cyclomethicone, or "polysiloxane."

---

### CLOGGED DRAINS
**What Your Thinning Hair Might Be Trying To Tell You**

We are going to resist the urge to play doctor here and say this: if you are a woman and you are losing your hair in clumps or at least notice more than a few strays in the shower, you should see a doctor. (And please, step away from the box of hair loss shampoo. If it worked, every man would be using it.) Female hair loss could be simply an unfortunate genetic drag—and not just from your mother's side, by the way; that's a myth.[10] Or, it could be that you have low iron, acute stress, polycystic ovarian syndrome, thyroid disease, lupus, or be exhibiting signs of premature menopause.[11] If you like your primary care doctor or dermatologist, you can try them first, or head straight for an endocrinologist, who tends to take anything hormone-related seriously from the first visit. It could be something beyond your control, or your body might be trying to tell you something. As always, you are advised to give her your ear.

---

## Treatments for Dandruff (and Other Scalp Problems)

Many **dandruff shampoos** contain coal tar—a known carcinogen. Regardless of what concentration levels may be deemed acceptable by the industry, we think it's best to skip it. Another common active ingredient in dandruff shampoos is zinc pyrithione, an ingredient that's proven to be toxic in animals, and more recently shown to cause real damage to human skin cells when applied topically.[12] Hmm. Here's our opinion on the matter: harsh products—many of which cause mild allergic reactions and exacerbate dryness—may be at the root of your flakes.

Of course, it's important to realize, too, that not all scalp issues are the same. Your scalp may be too dry, or producing too much sebum; you may also suffer from psoriasis, an autoimmune skin disorder that can be aggravated by stress, as well as external factors such as extreme heat, cold, and overwashing.[13] Whatever the cause, we suggest you start by switching to a super clean shampoo, and try alternating your washing with baking soda rinses, as baking soda is an effective antifungal.[14] One friend (with a buzz cut, granted) finally opted for the no-shampoo route after much coaxing; within a week his chronic scalp psoriasis had greatly improved. Another found that just switching from her chemical hair ingredients to clean ones made all the difference.

If you're brave enough to give yourself **scalp massages** with oils, as Rechelbacher recommends, we encourage that, too. Healthy plant oils have anti-inflammatory properties, and you can mix in some tea tree oil, which is also effective in the treatment of fungal and bacterial infections.[15] Including the right oils in your diet is key to fighting these skin conditions as well—you have our permission to skip ahead to Chapter 9 if you aren't familiar with the best internal anti-inflammatory foods and supplements. There's no time like the present to get your omega-3s.

## Straighteners, Relaxers, Keratin Treatments, and Perms

We understand that most women wage daily battles with their hair. Straight-haired girls wish they had beach-perfect waves, and curlies dream of sleek-straight tresses. Bless you if you've embraced yours, but we completely empathize if you have not. We also understand that societal mores favor long, silky-straight hair. At the end of the day, though, when we fight nature, nature tends to bite us in the ass in the form of chemical burns, drab and brittle strands that crack in half—that kind of thing.

We've already covered so-called **keratin treatments**, so we'll be brief. These contain keratin and a mystery blend of chemicals and sometimes even formaldehyde. (Ours sure did.) This mixture is flat-ironed onto your hair, "sealing" the hair while emitting noxious gases into the air for you and your stylist to inhale. It's expensive, it smells bad, and it's dangerous. We recounted our experience to Dr. Joseph Schwarcz, who is of the general perspective that women's exposure to chemicals in low doses through beauty products is not something we should be losing sleep over. But when we told him about our eye-burning, throat-aching reactions to this keratin treatment, he said, "There's just no way that you should be tearing up during a hair treatment. And, yes, that is a reaction to the formaldehyde."

As it turns out, some of these treatments contain more than ten times the amount of formaldehyde recommended by the CIR, which is not exactly known for being conservative in its recommendations. We say that if you are going for so much as a trim in a salon that offers this treatment, ask for an appointment when the service is not being performed. Yeah, that's a little high-maintenance and awkward, but it beats getting sick because someone else wanted to fork over $300-plus for six weeks of frizz-free hair. Pregnant? Find a new salon, mama.

**Chemical straighteners** and **relaxers** are no less kind. They actually break the chemical bonds that form curls in the first place, which is damaging to your hair. To accomplish this feat, cocktails of acids, sodium hydroxide, polyethylene glycol, propylene glycol, alcohols, and triethanolamine are employed.[16] A big problem with relaxers is they're usually used repeatedly, for years if not decades, which means your exposure to this scary combination is pretty much unrelenting. The toll these in-dividual chemicals take are bad enough as it is—not to men-tion the potential side effects of your hair falling out, unsightly chemical burns, eye damage, and allergic reactions—but how do they interact together? Well, that's the rub, ladies. We don't know. But our spidey sense tells us that if the ingredients are bad for you on their own, they probably don't play nice to-gether, either.

Onto **perms**. Perms, that '80s staple, are back! Which is bad news for our bodies. Briefly, creating curls requires a mélange of SLS, ethanolamine, borax, and the particularly problematic thioglycolic acid. Thioglycolates are toxic and have been known to cause low blood sugar (in case you've forgotten these things can get into your body), allergic reactions, foot swelling, and irreversible hair damage.[17]

Okay, shock therapy is over for now. Allow us to finish by saying if at all possible stop using chemicals to turn your hair into something it's not. Instead, go for less permanent versions of hair abuse. If you want your hair straight, use a gentle high-quality iron on a low setting, set aside a decent amount of time to do it properly, and then shower with a shower cap for a few days. Use dry shampoo if you get greasy. If you want curls, ditto. Just think of it as role playing: one day you're the wild, curly girl, and the next, you're that sleek sophisticate. The men (or women) in your life will thank you later.

## Dyes

First, the bad news: the FDA doesn't really regulate hair dyes. The EPA, meanwhile, claims that 69 percent of the dyes they've tested contained cancer-causing ingredients. An unscientific survey says what your gut probably does, too: the better the dyes work, the worse they are for you.

Slow down, though. Chemicals, yes. But whether those—or any of our beauty-product chems—cause cancer is still up for debate. The most recent definitive study by the International Agency for Research on Cancer (IARC) concluded that salon workers exposed to hair dyes that are "probably carcinogenic to humans" may increase risk of developing cancer over time.

We always think that when in doubt, consult Dr. Andrew Weil, health guru to millions. He had this to say on his website: "In general, I discourage use of hair dyes containing artificial coloring agents, which to my mind are as suspect in cosmetic products as they are in food. Hair dyes applied to the head are absorbed through the scalp, where there's a very rich blood supply that may carry them throughout the body. I'm sure that the new IARC report won't be the last word on this subject."

Other than delicately spraying fresh lemon juice on your hair or giving yourself an espresso rinse once in a while, we're going to refrain from recommending that you dye your hair. Natural dyes are available but are generally inconsistent in formulation, too chemically unreliable, and too terrible looking for us to recommend in good conscience. Meanwhile, the chemical-filled crap that actually looks good is really bad for you.

Of course, many of us don't want to go gray—though we'd love to see more people do it with pride—and some of us just love our highlights. Read "Siobhan's Tries to Detox Her Highlights" to get an idea of what expensive fancy salons do to your hair when you try to dye "naturally" and how she hasn't abandoned dyeing altogether.

If you also aren't ready to live without dye, then pick your battles, eat your broccoli, and keep your ear to the ground for more research on the matter.

## SIOBHAN TRIES TO DETOX HER HIGHLIGHTS

My colorist, Seth Silver, is a funny guy. He's as down-to-earth and non-judgmental as they come, but he also says things like, "Your natural hair color is never as nice as you think." But there are exceptions, I tell him. The girl born with the gorgeous deep chestnut; the cute redhead with those auburns everyone tried to copy in the '90s; that wheaty blonde with the (natural) locks I've been trying to nail for years.

It seems that most women think like Seth, though: a whopping 70 percent of us dye our hair—and you'd better believe most of us aren't using henna. More power to that 30 percent, but there's growing concern about what the rest of us should and shouldn't be doing in the name of beauty. Taking yet another cue from the Europeans, consider this: in 2006, the European Commission banned twenty-two ingredients to protect consumers from the potentially bladder-cancer-causing carcinogens in dyes. Twenty-two ingredients, I should add, that are all over the market this side of the pond.

So what has a decade of on-again-off-again highlighting done to me? Well, when Jackie O. died of cancer, some scientists blamed her years of bottled brown. Were they right? Who knows. But with that in mind, I thought it was high time I try something new. I'd heard about these gentler highlights that, while not chemical-free, are free of ammonia, lead, coal tar, and other carcinogens. It would be much, much gentler on my hair, on my bloodstream, and on the planet.

I'm one to try just about anything once, so I duck out of work one day to a salon that specializes in organic everything. The place is wind-powered. The people working there are charmingly bohemian without being crunchy. It seems like a sure bet, even if I know there's no such thing as truly organic, risk-free hair dye.

My new colorist is very pretty. She also has very pretty hair. She tells me she tries to eat vegan and wields a paintbrush in a way just casual enough to put me at ease. On my head, she will paint what will be, I'm certain, perfect, gentle blondes—as natural-looking as a little girl's, seamlessly blended with the dark blonde hair that actually grows out of my head. My new highlights will wash well, wear well, fade in the best way, and last longer than the ones I used to get years ago at the fancy department-store penthouse uptown. They won't be better than Seth's, but they'll be close. Of course they will.

At the salon, I'm struck by the smell—or lack thereof. There are no wafts of eye-burning ammonia. No itching at my temples. If this works, I think, womankind will rejoice: they'll be able to have the hair color they want, without the scary cancer-causing chems. As for me, I'm their willing and cheerful guinea pig.

But the second the foils come off, it hits me. *Oh. Crap. Ohcrap. Oh crapohcrapohcrap. Maybe it'll look better in natural light,* I tell myself. *Sure it will. This is natural, and natural always equals better. I just need to get this dried nice and quick and get out of here and check it with my compact mirror around the block. It'll be amazing.*

It was awful. I was sporting a horrible mess of splotchy stripes, as though the color hadn't set evenly. Or maybe it had, and it was just really ugly. Either way, it would have to be fixed. With my tail between my legs, off I went to Seth, who noticed and—bless his heart—*noted* the stripes at "hello." After I apologized for cheating on him, he smiled. "We'll fix you up. Don't worry," he said. With chemicals, mind you.

Since then, I still haven't fully given up dyeing my hair, but I've dialed down my highlight habit significantly. We do fewer pieces that last way longer, and we even things out with semi-permanent, low-tox toners in the gradual shift back to my natural color. Sure, I have a crisis of conscience every time I go see him (albeit a minor one), but for now have accepted it as the last bastion of my chemical romance. And when I walk by those unattractive green boxes of henna at the health food store, I think about it. Will I do it? Maybe next time.

## THE HAIR GUIDE

*Shampoo You Can Buy*

*Aubrey's Rosa Mosqueta Nourishing Shampoo*
How can you not trust a man who learned how to make natural cosmetics from his mother when he was nine. On a farm. In Indiana. There's a shampoo for every head in his line, but this is the best for color-treated hair of any we tried. Super shine-boosting and easy to rinse out. A dime size is plenty.

*Dr. Hauschka Shampoo with Apricot and Sea Buckthorn*
We don't know what sea buckthorn is, either, but we trust Dr. H. This shampoo is for dry and damaged hair, which we figure is almost everyone. The apricot along with the oil blends also mean it smells amazing, but not health-food-store amazing.

*CTonics Passion Shampoo*
*Elle* magazine named this the best green shampoo in 2009, and with good reason. This product is especially recommended for people with finer hair that has a tendency to frizz—though frankly, we think it's suitable for most hair types. Incredibly gentle, and so nourishing that it can also be used as a hair treatment that you leave in for a few minutes before rinsing.

*John Masters Organics Zinc and Sage Shampoo
with Conditioner*
For our money, this isn't really a two-in-one, though it is a lovely shampoo. It is extra-brightening for color-treated hair, and the

coconutty smell drives men insane. Expensive, but worth it as a weekly or biweekly rinse. Also good for sensitive scalps.

*Alaffia Coconut and Shea Butter Daily Shampoo*
Often available for less than ten bucks, this is a fantastic, nourishing shampoo for everyday use. It also smells incredible and uses fairly traded shea.

## Shampoo You Can Make

*Baking Soda Shampoo*
There's nothing that baking soda can't do. And when you dilute a tablespoon or so in a cup of water and cover your hair with it in the shower (making very sure that you then rinse it out), you'll get rid of dirty build-up without drying your hair out.

*Lemon or Apple Cider Vinegar Rinse*
These two natural cleansers also feature pH levels almost identical to conditioner, so you can do this rinse after shampoo or on its own. Mix either the juice of one lemon or two tablespoons of ACV into about a cup of water and cover hair in the shower, combing it through. And yes, the vinegar smell *does* go away.

*Cornstarch Dry Shampoo*
In between blowouts, or for less frequent shampooers, dry shampoo is a boon. Avoid pricey, store-bought formulas and just sprinkle cornstarch on your roots. Let it sit and absorb oils for a few minutes, then brush or pat out the excess.

*Traditional Indian Hibiscus Wash*
Take several hibiscus flowers and blend them with enough water (or lemon, or apple cider vinegar) to make a paste. Then

massage it into your scalp and hair and let sit for ten to fifteen minutes. Rinse thoroughly, and ta-da: super soft, shiny hair.

## Conditioner You Can Buy

*John Masters Honey and Hibiscus Hair Reconstructor*
Masters, a self-proclaimed "basement alchemist," has been at the chem-free game for decades. This conditioner smells incredible and somehow coats the hair shaft without weighing it down. Masters also cleverly uses moisture-retaining hyaluronic acid, which softens and seems to plump. It's a cult favorite.

*Aubrey's GPB Glycogen Protein Balancing Conditioner*
This pairs well with Aubrey's shampoo listed earlier, but we tried it on its own and it worked great, too. Made with coconut and aloe, it's extremely rich and not recommended for people prone to grease. Awesome on curls.

*John Masters Organics Lavender and Avocado Intensive Conditioner*
It doesn't have that old-lady lavender smell, and it smoothes without getting greasy the next day. It's great for air-drying waves and doesn't weigh down your hair.

*Intelligent Nutrients Leave-In Conditioner*
Both of us love this stuff. Again, it smells incredible. It offers wonderful control on curly hair and has a texturizing and volumizing effect on straight. It's also so clean you can eat it (though it's best you not try). Our only complaint? We wish there were more in every bottle.

## WHERE TO SHOP

When it comes to natural beauty, we really have to take our hats off to Whole Foods. It has done an excellent job at stocking this section of its stores—and its standards for choosing products are pretty stringent. With nearly three hundred locations in the United States, Canada, and Europe, it has made clean products a much more accessible commodity, and many of the items we suggest throughout the book can be found there.

If Whole Foods and natural food stores aren't your thing—or just aren't in your area—don't sweat it. As we were writing this book, it was pretty thrilling to see that the country's largest drugstore chains—Rite Aid, Target, CVS, and Walgreens—had started boasting "natural beauty" sections that feature some legitimate and well-priced clean products. Of course, even when so-called naturals are merchandised separately, distinguishing between the real cleans (or clean-enoughs) and the total fakers requires a close-read of ingredients. To simplify this process for you, at the end of each of our guides we will feature good products that you will likely find at the drugstore.

*Amazon Beauty Rahua Conditioner*
What's rahua, you ask? Why, it's a magical nut from deep in the Amazon, containing oil that will make your hair gorgeous, of course. Lore aside, this a great conditioner, and this company is doing good work with the women it employs in the Amazon and surrounding communities. There's also a leave-in treatment and an elixir.

## HOW TO WASH YOUR HAIR

If you're feeling adventurous, revisit "Wash Your Hair Backward" earlier in the chapter. Otherwise, here are some basic tips on cleaning your hair with clean products.

- Use only a quarter-size dollop of clean shampoo and understand it will not foam the way your old shampoo does.
- Lather it up in your hands with a little water.
- Run your hands over your roots. The ends will get cleaned as it rinses out of your hair.
- Rinse well.
- Put a dollop of clean conditioner the size of quarter to two quarters in your hand and smooth over your hair, starting at the root, all the way down to the tip.
- If you feel like it, comb it through to distribute it evenly.
- Leave the conditioner in for a couple of minutes. If you're using a clean conditioner, you won't get greasy, we promise. Do something else, like shave your legs, in the meantime.
- Rinse thoroughly.
- Towel dry your ends gently, and avoid turbaning your hair.
- Apply any styling aid you like.
- Comb through.
- Dry or air dry as usual.

## Conditioner You Can Make

### Mayonnaise Mask

Obviously, we're talking the organic kind, or just make it yourself with eggs and olive oil. Use a tablespoon or two on its own, add lemon juice, or go halfsies with an avocado. Leave it in for however long you can stand it (forty minutes at the most).

### Avocado Mask

When God created food. . . . Avocado is so packed with good stuff, you could probably just live on it and never lack in nutrients. Just mash it up, leave it in—again, it can be used on its own or combined with other ingredients on this list. Don't forget to eat your leftovers; internal benefits abound.

### Coconut Milk Rinse

Yes there's a theme on this list: fats and proteins. All things coconut can be used in hair, though the milk has the best consistency as a conditioner. The oil is nice, too, and can penetrate the cuticle to fortify the inside part of your hair. Throw on some reggae, and try it with the avocado. Just kidding.

### Carrier Oil Treatments

We like jojoba, olive, coconut, and sweet almond for hair. After saturating your hair in as much as a quarter cup, which you could even leave on overnight if you don't mind sleeping with a plastic bag around your head, try doing a baking soda rinse to get rid of any excess.

## Styling Products You Can Buy

### John Masters Organics Shine On

This is good for super dry or shorter styles, because it's a tad rich. Most shine serums use silicone to coat your locks without nourishing them. JMO, of course, would never do that to us.

HAIR

Instead, he uses moisture- and shine-boosting kelp and fagus sylvaticus extract. (That's Latin for awesome.)

### Simply Organic Medium Hold Hair Spray

We'll keep this reminder brief: conventional hair spray can give you babies who pee up instead of down. Don't use it. This stuff is one of the few naturals that actually holds well, washes out easily, and doesn't smell funny.

### Aubrey's Mandarin Magic Ginkgo Leaf and Ginseng Root Hair Jelly

Name's a mouthful, but it works like a charm. We can't help but notice that two of the first three ingredients are basically free and easy to use on your own (water? aloe?), but they make up for it with thickening natural gums that soften and thicken your hair as it holds. Plus it's low-shine, so you won't look like That Girl.

### Intelligent Nutrients Everything

We're obsessed with the volumizing spray. It lifts at the roots, adds a nice texture, and stays put for hours without being crunchy. We also really like IN's finishing gloss, and if you're a gel gal, there's a good one here, too. Pretty much this line does no wrong, so try your particular product-type preference.

### Aloe Vera Everything

If you're going to read only one paragraph in this section, make it this one, because aloe vera is a hair care godsend. It's like a ten-in-one for all your hair concerns. Shine? Check. Frizz? Check. Hold, curl, moisture? Yup. Its high-sulphur and slightly acidic pH make it a natural antibacterial (great for

HAIR

---

## YOUR HAIR AT THE DRUGSTORE

Many drugstores are now carrying the **Giovanni** hair care line. This is a great brand to start your new routine with: it feels and smells remarkably like the mainstream products you're used to (including a wide array of styling products), but with much cleaner ingredients and great prices. Another good option for conditioner is the now widely available **Yes To** line (which includes Yes To Carrots, Yes To Tomatoes, and Yes To Cucumbers), but we do not recommend the shampoo because it contains sulfates. Take note, too, that there is fragrance in their formulation; so while we don't endorse that choice, the overall ingredients list is still far cleaner than the average product. **Burt's Bees**, while not our favorite for hair (though we really love some of their other stuff), is also now a drugstore mainstay, if you're in a pinch. Other cleaner hair brands we've come across: **E-sen-cia** and **Avalon Organics**.

---

dandruff) and style product, but because it's 99 percent water, it's not astringent enough to overdry. If you're curly or have thinner hair, go for pure aloe in liquid form, and put it in a spray bottle with half a teaspoon of whatever oil you like. Still not sold? It's the active botanical in more "natural" styling products than we can name, ladies. So cut out the middle man. Stock up on the stuff.

*Flax Seed Gel*

Boil one or two tablespoons of ground flaxseeds in a cup of water to create a frothy gel-like consistency that makes for a nice, strong hold-and-shine as a hair gel. Versatile and rich in omega-3s, which encourage hair growth, it's what Aveda and others use in their products, and what flappers used in the '20s for that pin-curl look.

### Lemon Vodka Hair Spray

There are lots of recipes out there for homemade hair sprays, but this is our favorite. You're going to want to simmer three sliced lemons in water for thirty minutes on low. The vodka is optional, but it works as a good preservative, which means you can make it—and keep it around—in batches.

### Egg White Mousse

If you want to add volume at your roots, try a bit of cornstarch on dry hair. If you're dead-set on mimicking mousse's actual consistency, though, you're going to need to go meringue. Froth up about four egg whites and put 'em in your hair. It holds surprisingly well, but it's certainly not vegan, and it's certainly not for everyone.

# 5

## Your Face

If we lived on a desert island without makeup, pollution, and dates, we probably wouldn't wash our faces much. We might splash with some seawater now and again, then crack the occasional coconut for a soothing rinse, but we'd do that because it feels nice, not because we're obsessed with the idea of being clean. It wasn't always so—we used to foam and scrub and peel like the best of them. That is, until we learned that we might be creating more problems than we were solving.

Ever met someone who says they don't wash their face at all? Us, too. We've even had boyfriends like this, and looking at their near-perfect complexions sort of made us want to cry. Did they not wash their face because they had perfect skin to begin with, or did not using gobs of cleanser every day allow a natural glory to reveal itself? Impossible to know, but instinct tells us that before the advent of modern cosmetics chemistry, people's complexions were probably a lot more balanced than they are now—even if they didn't have the helpful anti-aging marvels we'll get into a little later. Truth be told, our skin probably wouldn't need as much maintenance if we weren't always putting dirty, pore-clogging things on it. But we do, and so we do.

## MEET YOUR FACE

The top layer of your skin has something called an acid mantle on it: made up of sweat and oil, this is our first defense against the elements and things like bacteria and fungal infections. Before puberty, our skin is more alkaline, making young people more prone to infection and illness; as we hit adolescence, it starts to protect us; but since most things eventually cycle back to their beginnings, we lose it again as we get older. But we're not there yet, so most of us should have skin with a pH around 5.5—slightly acidic. In order to rid it of the pollution, makeup, oil, dead skin cells, and other daily debris, you probably use something highly alkaline, like soap or some other cleanser that makes you feel squeaky-clean. (That feeling isn't actually what's best for you—as you've probably guessed by now.) Most soaps have a pH around 10, which launches your skin in the other direction—that's why it feels so different after you wash it.

There are competing theories about how good or bad alkaline soaps are for the skin, and whether or not you need to restore pH with a toner after you wash to get your skin back to "normal," or not disrupt it at all by using low-pH cleansers in the first place, yadda-yadda. The bottom line is that modern living necessitates face washing, but you *can* wash without disrupting the acid mantle, without unwittingly causing breakouts, and without ushering in toxic chemicals you do not want in your body in the first place. Let's talk about how.

## Cleansers

When you're choosing a cleanser, you want to go gentle. For those of you with sensitive or mature skin, you know from experience that washing can stress out your already delicate dermis, robbing you of the oils and plumpness that make you glow. For those with super active skin—inflamed, irritated, or acne-prone—you so much as splash your face, and something unexpected can happen: a rashy reaction to some ingredient, the revelation of a zit, or splotchy patches you now have to hide under makeup. But even girls blessed with more even-keeled complexions may be doing hidden harm with their face wash.

The first problem with most cleansers is that they're too harsh—even if the bottle claims "gentle" or "hypoallergenic" or "non-comedogenic." Some of the "gentlest" cleansers we reviewed contained the harshest detergent on the market, not to mention silicones, dyes, and no fewer than four chemical preservatives.

As we explained with shampoos—you'd be surprised how much your shampoo and face wash have in common—sulfates are surfactants used in many cleansers, and in addition to being drying and irritating, they also might be contaminated with a carcinogen called 1,4-dioxane. Surfactants are wetting agents that bind to oil and debris and wash them away, so you can understand why so many companies use them. In the simplest of terms, they are effective—but they're not really doing what's ideal. You want something to gently remove the *excess* oil and the dirt, without compromising your skin's natural balance.

Which brings us to penetration enhancers. These are popular in cleansers, and for the life of us we cannot understand why.

In washing the surface of your face, no one wins when that stuff gets deep into your pores—not even if you have acne; that's what treatment products are for. You know, the ones you leave on long enough to work. (And if it is powerful enough to get deep into your pores in the thirty seconds it takes to wash your face, it's probably extremely harsh and therefore unkind to your skin in other ways.) To avoid these, check the label for ingredients that are known to penetrate, such as acids, PEGs, sulfates, and propylene glycol.

Another no-no in cleansers is artificial fragrance. As we've explained, these are chemical compounds made up of countless mysterious ingredients, many of which are skin irritants or, worse, hormone disruptors. Here's the reality about fragrances in cleansers: they're there to trick you into thinking that you're using something special, when really you're using something nearly identical to the last thing you bought. There is no good reason for your face to go to the perfume counter every day.

Many experts we trust advise a simple olive- or coconut-oil-based bar soap with as few ingredients as possible—like, two or three. Any health food and many grocery stores will have a few options for less than four bucks that will last you months. Just be diligent about checking for fragrance: it should not have any, and if it does, make sure it identifies the source of the scent. Bar soaps will have a higher pH, if you are concerned about such things. If it feels good, great. If your skin is taut after washing, rather than double up on moisturizer, try something gentler.

There is a school of thought that disrupted pH is the cause of some acne and premature aging. If you want to tackle that one, or if you simply prefer the feeling of a nonfoaming cleanser, go for a gel or milky one. Bear in mind, however, that if you are using a liquid, you are probably exposing yourself to even more ingredients, which means even more can go wrong. Traditional cleansers, both foaming and not, might pack in sulfates, triethanolamine, parabens, alcohol, fragrance, propylene glycol, and others. You may recognize a few of those from our dirty ingredient list in Chapter 3, and none of them will make your skin look nice.

No cleanser will perform miracles, but when you use a gentle one, your skin loves you back by looking dewy and supple. We like nonfoaming cleansers from Evan Healy, Dr. Hauschka, and Ren. They're all pH compatible with skin and work well on a variety of skin types. They're not inexpensive, though. For more about these and some more affordable ones, check our guide at the end of the chapter.

And listen, we understand the temptation to have a treatment-oriented regimen, but washing your face isn't supposed to do a whole lot more than, well, wash your face. It can't take ten years off your life or cure your acne. While a few soothing active ingredients such as calendula or chamomile in your cleanser, or tea tree oil as an antibacterial aren't bad ideas, you are probably better off saving these special ingredients for products that stay *on* your face. Otherwise, it's down the drain it goes—along with your hard-earned dollars.

## THE ART OF DOUBLE CLEANSING

There is another way to wash your face that beauty insiders swear by. They will cross themselves up and down, promising that it cleared their mild acne, took years off their faces, and helped them maintain an even, dewy complexion. If you have relatively cooperative skin, we highly recommend you try this method.

(For really temperamental skin, or in cases of cystic acne deep below the surface, we *do not* recommend this method. It might be a case of getting much worse before it gets much better, but we're not about to ask you to sit around as your skin performs an opera right there on your face.)

So, here's how it works. Start by picking an organic oil that you like. Coconut is a favorite, but make sure it's raw and cold pressed; other people like olive—the same guidelines apply. Organic matters here because you don't want to be massaging pesticides into your face. Put a little oil in the palm of your dry hand and, using your fingertips, slowly massage it into your skin using a downward circular motion. If you're feeling rich, add a little steam to the routine, or lay a warm washcloth over your face.

After a couple of minutes, grab your natural, nonirritating cleanser and wash off the residue, concentrating on areas prone to breakouts, like the T-zone. There. You're done. The first time you do this, you will probably be pretty freaked out. We know putting oil on your face is counterintuitive. You may also get a few little whiteheads a day or two after. This is not a bad sign. It means debris under the skin has been loosened and has decided it is ready to present itself to the world. It sucks, but they do stop coming, and what is left is glowy, lovely, balanced skin.

## Toners and Astringents

Back in the day, we thought we were so savvy. We didn't buy into that heavily marketed three-part system prescription. We'd look at an expensive bottle of toner and think, "What do you take us for, morons? Twenty bucks for a bottle of water, and alcohol you can't even drink?" Our instincts weren't all wrong: most toners suck. But in an ironic twist, we've come to embrace this product category, which indeed serves a purpose after all—first though, a look at the bad ones.

The main ingredients in most of these products are water and alcohol. Water is free from your tap, and alcohol can be extremely drying. To counter the drying effects of too much alcohol, companies will throw in some soothers, skin conditioning agents, dyes to make the product look nice, synthetic stench, and preservatives. Targeted ones might contain salicylic acid, the beta hydroxy acid that is considered effective in the treatment of pimples, but which in high doses can be toxic.[1]

We have grown to appreciate other toners, however. We might even say we're a little obsessed. These can be especially useful in the application of moisturizers and face oils, because their water content combines with the rich oils in topicals to mimic the skin's natural composition. Another benefit is their use after a particularly alkaline cleansing. A pH-balancing toner can help restore your skin to what it was like before you washed it. This is a less convincing argument to us (again, see the desert-island fantasy), but there's something to the science.

If you're game, here's how you use it: when you're done washing your face, pat dry and then spritz your face with a toner immediately before you moisturize. A lot of the treatment toners out there also do the job of rationing some good ingredients for your skin that might be irritating in higher concentrations. For people with acne, you can try one with the natural salicylic acid, or even better, tea tree oil, as well as something soothing like chamomile or calendula to beat out redness and inflammation. For anti-aging, green tea's a good bet, as is anything containing other A-team antioxidants that we'll list later on.

Certain holistic skin care gurus swear by the almost miraculous healing powers of hydrosols, which are basically the water that remains after oils are distilled from their source. Evan Healy makes lovely ones, as does Elisha Reverby, whose boutique line Elique Organics has become a beauty insider's secret weapon of choice. Both women are lifelong studiers of skin care and beauty chemistry and know of what they speak. They advise spritzing right before moisturizing (or even mixing the two in your hand). Do it on planes, before bed, after lunch, on your baby—there are no rules with these truly clean flower waters.

Another useful trick is to use a spritz toner to set your mineral makeup. Anyone who's played around with powders knows how chalky they can look on a bad day or if applied in a hurry. Here, just lightly mist your powder-finished face and then leave it alone. It imparts a dewiness to the look without making you shiny.

## Acne Treatments

We're going to be brief here because it's our opinion—and that of countless experts—that acne is something that should be treated internally, through supplements, food, and hormone regulation. Topicals should just be pinch-hitting as needed. People like to talk about a special kind of skin problem called hormonal acne, but the truth is that all acne is hormonal—it just varies from person to person which hormone is doing the damage. Cortisol, the stress hormone, can send a cascade of oil out of your sebaceous glands when you're panicky. Testos-

terone and "male" hormones can cause women to overproduce
sebum, whereas too much estrogen and too much T4 are aggra-
vators as well. Because acne is an inflammatory disease, flare-
ups can be triggered by all kinds of other things as well (see
Chapter 9 for more about this), including the harsh ingredients
in the topicals used to get rid of zits in the first place.

**Benzoyl peroxide** (BP) is the most popular over-the-
counter treatment for acne in the United States, and it's a
beast. It is able to reach and kill bacteria through hair follicles;[2]
it's also been banned for use in Europe. It appears that those
Europeans may have been put off by the link between BP and
cancer: studies indicate that it is a free-radical-generating compound, shown to promote tumors in mice when applied topically.[3] Topically, ladies—like the cream we all used at one time
or another. As you may have guessed, "free-radical-generating"
does not bode well for skin aging either; topical application in
mice showed it to "qualitatively resemble" the effects of UVB
rays. Making matters worse, it's most effective in acne treatment when it's used in some kind of treatment that stays on the
skin (though it still appears in cleansers and scrubs for marketing purposes). In creams, it's paired with familiar baddies like
PEGs, propylene glycol (which probably helps it penetrate),
parabens, and other less familiar ingredients. BP boasts other
skills on its résumé, as well—such as bleaching fabric on contact and being an explosive.[4]

**Tea tree oil** is considered the gold standard natural alternative to BP. It is a natural antiseptic, antifungal, and antibiotic
that has been shown to be useful in beating out dandruff, scary
infections like MRSA, and your trusty zits.[5] In fact, one study
even showed that applying a tea tree oil gel with 5 percent concentration was as effective as a benzoyl peroxide solution of

the same concentration. It showed a slightly slower zit-banishing power, but on the plus side, it triggered fewer side effects (like flaky red skin).[6] Considering what happens to the dermis whenever we've used BP, anything as effective and less aggressive sounds like a good call to us. If you do use tea tree oil, go easy, though. One drop, diluted in your face cream or another oil, is more than enough. (We have found it works on cold sores, too.)

**Salicylic acid** is the other go-to topical in conventional zit zappers. Burt's Bees recently isolated it at its natural source, in willow bark, and has developed a mostly natural line of skin care built around it. It attacks acne on multiple fronts—it's exfoliating, functions as an antimicrobial, and, being from the aspirin family, it's also an anti-inflammatory.[7] Categorized as a beta hydroxy acid, it is both gentler than alphahydroxy and better at penetrating pores, making it pretty effective on blackheads *and* whiteheads. But it's still an acid, and we have reservations about them: they can be dehydrating, aggravating, and disrupt the skin's natural balance. In other bad news, salicylic acid is verboten for pregnant women, as it is a documented teratogen—it can produce birth defects.[8] What does that mean for those of us not currently knocked up? Good question. Salicylic acid also has a well-documented history of transdermal poisoning. At its most dramatic—used at a 20 percent concentration and over a large area of the body—it killed two people.[9] Is this a real case of the dose makes the poison? Possibly. But, as usual, we don't see the point of putting that unnecessary strain on our body. If you're already devoted to it, then try the Burt's Bees line to ensure an overall cleaner product.

For ages, **sulphur** was hailed a zit-stopper, and it still pops up in cult hits from Kate Sommerville and Mario Badescu. The science here is a little confusing. On the one hand, it was shown to have good bacteria-killing and oil-soaking abilities. But, on the flip side, research in the 1970s seemed to suggest that, in fact, sulphur might be comedogenic—derm speak for pore-clogging. In a study called "Is Sulphur Helpful or Harmful in Acne Vulgaris?" published in 1972, sulphur was found to be both. Creams containing elemental sulphur were actually shown to cause pimples on the human back when applied, leading researchers to surmise that regular use of the stuff might perpetuate, rather than fix, acne: it would dry out the zit on the surface, while clogging up the skin beneath, causing more pimples. Here's what we think: on a regular, not-too-deep zit, it dries them off overnight, but don't go using this stuff every night, and be sure to wash your face well in the morning.

## WASHING WITH STICKS
### And Siobhan's Other Creative Attempts to Banish Breakouts

As I'm packing my suitcase for a yoga ashram, two things occur to me. First, because of the new skin care regimen prescribed by a stern Ayurvedic doctor named Pratima Raichur, I will not have to check any luggage. The centerpiece of my new, twice-daily cleansing ritual is a bottle of what looks like crushed up sticks (just add water). Second, I am almost certainly becoming That Girl. The one who goes to the ashram to get away from her stress-and-zit-ridden life in the big city with magical Indian tinctures and powders in hand.

It had been a rough couple of months, fueled by too much travel, too much socializing, and too much work, and my skin was letting me have it. In addition to the hormonal zits many of us battle monthly, I also had a mysterious, prickly rash on my upper chest, and these

sticks—followed by natural antibacterial neem oil and some supplements—were going to get my skin in check.

Given Pratima's cult status among celebrities (as well as girls I know
and trust), I was willing to give this my all. Neem, I already knew, has
well-documented powers over pests of all kinds: insects, bacteria, fungus. It's not the most pleasant smelling stuff in the world, but I'd been
told it works, and that was what we were going for. As if by magic, after a week of diligently following her instructions, washing with a
mélange of dried sandalwood, neem, and cooling coriander and then
massaging with pure neem oil, my skin rewarded me. It wasn't perfect,
but it was close. All the inflammation was gone, along with the stress
cycle it helped perpetuate.

The truth is, acne is hormonal, and you can try as best you can to
control those hormones, get them in check by reducing stress, avoiding sugar, flushing out excess androgens with prescriptions like
spironolactone, or taking birth control pills, but we are fickle beasts.
Sometimes our bodies cooperate, and sometimes, especially when it
comes to breakouts, they do not.

As a result, in between ashram visits I've been known to try just
about anything, from crunchy naturals to caustic synthetics. During another bad skin spell, I paid a visit to the dermatologist Dr. Doris Day.
Aside from having the best name and great skin, she's a mainstay in all
the women's magazines, dishing out no-bullshit advice about all our
pesky problems. She also takes acne very seriously, and seems to enjoy getting to the bottom of it (which is more than I can say about any
other dermatologist I've met—and I've met plenty).

She suggested I try a new treatment called Isolaz. Now here's the
thing with lasers: I know they aren't natural per se, but I'm into
proven, gentle, and safe skin care, and nonablative lasers sort of fit that
criteria. Isolaz was all over the press at the time, touted as one of the
more promising lasers for acne, so off I went. The procedure is simple:
a suction device cleans the skin of debris, then a rubber-band-snap of
laser zaps the bacteria. It doesn't hurt. It doesn't have any serious side
effects when done properly, and . . . it works.

Over several sessions, my skin improved considerably. My pores were clearer, smaller, and I had fewer zits—almost none in fact. People noticed something was different about my overall appearance, but couldn't identify what exactly. But here's the catch: once I stopped going, it was as if the skin gods were punishing me for trying to foil it with fancy lights and suction cups.

I haven't been to an ashram in a while, and I'm no longer washing with sticks, but my skin care regimen is completely natural and organic. I take four high-quality omega-3 capsules twice a day along with zinc and vitamin E, and my skin has been more cooperative than ever. I also try to keep my hormones in check with the help of my endocrinologist, stick to gentle cleansers and clays, *never* skimp on beneficial topical oils, and yup, I still hightail it to Dr. Day's office when things get really ugly.

## Exfoliating Scrubs

Step away from the crushed nuts—we need to talk real quick. People can't seem to agree on the relative merits of exfoliation. We will say for the record that we don't think these are necessary, and in fact they might be bad for us. See, nature has its logic. If there are dead skin cells on the surface of our skin, it's because nature wants to protect the more delicate skin beneath. Over time, these will slough off *on their own*, when they're good and ready. Physically scrubbing them off with anything other than a soft washcloth, meanwhile, can cause tiny tears in the skin, provoking inflammation, irritating acne and spreading around bacteria. We had a hard time finding any compelling expert advice that convinced us it was worth our money, or the health of our skin.

We have also found that since we changed the products we use, our skin has naturally just gotten more vibrant, less dull, and less prone to flakiness. (To that last point, if your skin is flaking off, you should figure out why, not just try to treat the flakes by scraping them off. It could be that your cleanser is too drying or that some other topical is irritating your skin.) But enough with the preaching. We know how delicious skin looks after a carefully done scrub with good ingredients, so even though we don't wholly advocate this, let's look at what makes a good one versus a bad.

You've probably caught on already that our tastes skew a little more natural, but here's where nature might fail you. Irregular and rough-cut particles can really do more harm than good by tearing and stripping the skin. (It feels good while you're scrubbing though, doesn't it?) On the flip side, jojoba beads are natural, as is finely ground oatmeal, and both make popular and effective alternatives. We've also experimented with pure baking soda, which you can use with water. Baking soda is pretty alkaline and can irritate redness-prone skin. Salt is another option, but it stings, and be careful with sugar and other things that bacteria like to feed on. While we think sugar can make for a nice body scrub, keep it away from any part of you that may break out.

Conventional scrubs, even the ones that seem natural, usually have a scrubby substance of some kind like apricot seeds or the aforementioned crushed nut shells, mixed with paraben preservatives, fragrance, PEGs, alcohol, and propylene glycol. You know the drill with these. An added precaution: since scrubbing can enhance the penetration of other things—both good and bad—you want to be extra careful of what's in these products, and what you pile on after.

## Chemical Exfoliants and Peels

Alphahydroxy acids (AHAs) are about as controversial as they are effective—which is to say, quite. They're used in a wide array of products in the mainstream and natural markets, and there are several different kinds, with different origins: lactic (milk), glycolic (sugar), citric (oranges and lemons), malic (apples and pears), and taratic (grapes). What they all have in common is their ability to burn off—"dissolve," if you prefer—the top layer of your skin in the right concentration. In low concentrations, AHAs can enhance moisture in the skin, because they work as a water-binding agent. In higher amounts they have been shown to reduce acne scars, undo the visible signs of sun damage, and increase the thickness of the skin beneath, resulting in a firmer appearance.[10] At first, this sounds like a total win-win.

Look into the safety of AHAs and you will see frequent mention of how Cleopatra used to bathe in lactic acid to make her skin nice, and how AHAs occur in nature—a convenient instance where the cosmetics industry touts "natural" as a good thing. Of course, not all things natural are good for us (see botulism) and, more important, not all things natural should be extracted from their source and applied to our skin in concentrated form. All that aside, though, 99 percent of the AHAs used in cosmetics are synthetic.[11]

AHAs have been on health watch lists for some time. There is plenty of evidence that AHAs increase sun sensitivity and cell damage from UV exposure.[12] There is also evidence that this increased risk goes away within a week of stopping AHA use. Because of the increased UV risk and the fact that AHAs can cause second-degree burns on the face and neck, the consensus in the business seems to be that AHAs are best used at home in concentrations of 10 percent or lower in a topical cream and in conjunction with a sunscreen.[13]

In 2007, the National Toxicology Program at the National Institutes of Health (NIH) produced a 244-page report where scientists used mice to assess skin-cancer risk with glycolic acid and salicylic acid. The FDA and the PCPC have had lots of back-and-forth on the matter as well; the CIR's Final Report positioned AHAs as safe when used by consumers in concentrations of 10 percent or lower, and up to 30 percent by estheticians for treatments and when sun-protection is also recommended.[14] As of 2005, the FDA has recommended (but not mandated) that AHA-containing products include a sunburn warning on the bottle.[15]

So where does that leave you? With a tricky decision to make. You'll find that these turn up low on the ingredient lists in a bunch of natural products. We don't have much of an issue with that. Know that using these might compromise the skin's natural barrier function, increase your risk of UV damage, increase absorption of things that don't belong in your body, and irritate your skin all at the same time. If you're going to read that and use products or peels containing acids anyway, pick one that plainly states its level of concentration on the bottle, use it only as directed—never more—and make sure you use broad-spectrum sunscreen at the same time. Juice Beauty and Arcona lead the way with their fruit-derived extracts. Or, opt for a pure clay mask, which imparts similar benefits without the acids.

## Moisturizers, Lotions, and Oils

As you'll probably recall, it's often not the active ingredients in a product you have to worry the most about: it's all the other crap. Let's separate our moisturizing friends from our foes, shall we?

Here's what moisturizers don't do: they do not enhance your skin's elasticity; they can't reverse sun damage; they can't make your wrinkles go away.[16] What they can do is attract and retain moisture in the outer layers of your skin and provide a protective film on its surface. This can have lots of beneficial cosmetic effects because it feels nice and can make the skin appear softer, smoother, and plumper since hydrated skin looks more youthful than dry skin. Given the number of promises out there about the miracles of moisturizers, that may seem like small potatoes, but it's not nothing.

When we moisturize, we are typically adding *humectants*, which help attract and retain moisture from inside and outside the skin; *emollients*, which are fats and oils; and *occlusives*. Petrolatum and other petrochemicals are widely used occlusives despite the fact that they are not considered safe by many experts and are byproducts of a decidedly unrenewable resource—maybe you didn't realize that we fight wars in the Middle East for moisturizer. These work by literally creating a film on top of the skin that stops moisture from evaporating out of the skin. (By sealing it, however, they also stop moisture from going in.) Because water originates in the deeper layers of skin, humectants draw the moisture to the surface, and occlusives keep them there. We appreciate the elegant chemistry and all, but there's got to be a better way to restore moisture balance in our skin. Here's a clue: stop dehydrating it in the first place, and then maybe you won't need to put Vaseline on it.

Moisturizers, which have to be stable in different conditions and last a long time in your humid bathroom (and on the drugstore shelf), tend to be loaded with preservatives and other chemicals. As with body lotion, face lotions deserve your attention because they are meant to sit on and in your skin for long periods of time without being washed off, they work best when they penetrate well, and are used often twice a day, every day, for decades. That's a lot of exposure to ingredients that might not be good for you. Many lotions include parabens or formaldehyde-releasing preservatives like DMDM hydantoin, as well as petrolatum or paraffin to seal moisture in the skin, triethanolamine and other pH adjusters or stabilizers, PEGs, and fragrance or fragrance maskers. What in that list says beautiful skin?

On the clean side, you'll find natural combinations of ingredients with similar functions. You still need to hydrate and soothe the skin, lock in or attract moisture, and make sure the bottle doesn't go rancid two weeks after you open it. But instead of petrolatum and emollients, you will find skin-friendly oils, purified water, aloe, and active extracts with (hopefully) proven therapeutic qualities to them.

For this reason and others, we've taken a shine to face oils. Contrary to what you'd think, using pure oils on your skin does not make your face look gross. In fact, we've found the opposite to be true: if you use a small amount, you get the glow of well-hydrated, gently taken care of skin without the shine or stickiness you get from certain lotions. Even better, most oils recommended for topical application on their own—like coconut, jojoba, olive, and newly popular argan—are not only exceptional moisturizers: they also double as SPF, and come equipped with their own anti-inflammatory and antioxidant properties.

One all-star oil, which you can use on its own or in a store-bought natural lotion as long as it's pretty high up on the ingredients list, is extra virgin olive oil (EVOO). In addition to packing antioxidants and skin-friendly fats, EVOO also enhances UVB protection when applied before sun exposure, and reduces sun damage when applied after.[17] If you're using this as your moisturizer, that's a pretty notable bonus, wouldn't you say? Especially if you consider that some contaminants in petrochemical-based moisturizers are known carcinogens. Take your pick: the possibly carcinogenic petrochem lotion, or cancer-fighting olive oil?

Spirit Demerson, who founded the luxurious online organic-skin care site Spirit Beauty Lounge, swears by iLA Face Oil. "Argan oil is really high in antioxidants, which is great for mature skin and dry skin, and the rosehip seed oil is an excellent hydrator and feels silky. These are rare and expensive, but with that you're going to get something that feels comparable to a department store cream in terms of luxuriousness and effectiveness, but the department store cream is 70 percent synthetic chemicals and water."

We do love us some argan oil. Not only is it an excellent hydrator, it's also loaded with the antioxidant vitamin E and linoleic acid, which work well together to beat off free radical damage, as well as all kinds of inflammation such as acne.[18] (The zit-afflicted swear by it; one study even showed it slowed sebum production.[19]) "I have always had difficult combination skin, very dry, but oily on my chin and forehead," says Katharine L'Heureux, whose Kahina Giving Beauty skin care line is built around this miraculous Moroccan oil. "Argan oil is the first thing that I have ever used that has balanced my skin. My skin is much softer and has a healthy glow. I am approaching fifty but have had crowsfeet since I was in my twenties. I have noticed these lines becoming minimized since using argan oil every night."

She's not alone. The legendary makeup artist Rose-Marie Swift uses it in her natural makeup line; and the model-cum-natural-beauty-magnate Josie Maran says it's her beauty secret, too. If you're not convinced, just look at a picture of Maran and her baby's-butt skin. The trick, of course, is to make sure the oil is organic, and then to leave the ingredient alone. "When I discovered argan, I thought, 'What a perfect, pure product,'" L'Heureux says. "I couldn't imagine polluting this clean ingredient with anything that was harmful, so I've tried to create a line that lives up to the standard of argan oil using all natural ingredients with a high percentage of organic botanicals." Maran sells an argan, too, that is clean and organic.

Of course, not every company is treating the ingredient this way. Its popularity means it's also being sprinkled into all kinds of mainstream commercial brands. Kiehl's, for example, has a capsule collection containing argan oil, but in most of the products, the argan oil is pretty far down on the ingredients list, beat out by sulfates, penetration enhancers, cheaper oils, and alcohol. This is a reminder to read ingredients and choose your products carefully.

In a clean moisturizer, you should look for actives that suit your skin type in a base made up of purified water, nutrient-rich oil like rosehip seed, olive, coconut or argan, shea butter, possibly aloe, and that's about it. The words will probably appear on labels in Latin—that's a good sign. On the other hand, chemical words with lots of "Xs" and "Ys" and "eths" and hyphens are code for "You do not want to buy me."

## Sunscreen

It should come as no surprise that we're about to tell you to use sunscreen. You can hem and haw, making valid claims about your need for vitamin D, how happy the beach makes you, and how gross the stuff feels on your face, but if you want to keep your skin looking as good as possible, sunscreen is a nonnegotiable. We'll talk later about vitamin D and how it's okay to get some unprotected rays on your body. But right now we're talking mugs, and if you love yours you will pay heed.

Back in Chapter 3 we told you about some of the concern surrounding chemical sunscreens, namely that PABA is a suspected carcinogen and that the very popular oxybenzone may be an endocrine disruptor that is showing up in everyone's pee, not to mention the environment (and possibly our water).[20] We also pointed out that the tricky tricksters who came up with the SPF rating are referring only to UVB rays, which is a mere half of the problem when it comes to protecting our skin from cancer and sun damage (SPF will protect you from sunburns though). What we didn't get to was all the other questionable ingredients in there.

We will revisit sunscreens in Chapter 7 and look at why slathering these chemicals from head to toe on repeat is not the best idea. Just from a vanity perspective, though, here are a few things that pop up in sunscreen that you don't want on your face: fragrance (for obvious reasons), alcohol (it dries), nanoparticles (because who knows what they're dragging in and where they're going), formaldehyde releasers (this does not need to be explained), and so on. Your typical sunscreen may have some or all of these ingredients. More dangerous still is the false sense of comfort sunscreens serve up.

So what to do? The easiest answer is to avoid sun exposure on your face: draw the blinds when there's direct light coming through (yes, UVA rays *do* penetrate glass); stay in the shade; and invest in a wide-brimmed hat. If that's crazy talk for you, then use some of our favorite broad-spectrum, clean sun-screens that use zinc and titanium dioxide and other face-friendly ingredients. Mineral makeup is also a good bet, since titanium dioxide or zinc are usually there in significant concentrations. However, if you're going to be spending real time in the sun, it's wise to layer them with a sunscreen too (cream first). If you're using only sunscreen, don't skimp—and reapply.

Note to girls with darker skin: if your skin is a deep, dark brown then, yes, it is true that it comes equipped with its own sun-filtering power (equivalent to about SPF 15). But it's a misconception to think that you're immune to the dangers and damages of the sun—including skin cancer, which though less common tends to be diagnosed at later more dangerous stages in people with darker skin. Hopefully you know this already. We understand, though, that some minerals can look slightly chalky or have a subtle matte finish, but good mineral makeup options are becoming more available for all complexions—like Alima—which we will cover more in Chapter 6.

## Anti-Agers

There's not much we women won't do to break free from the grip of Father Time. It's no surprise, then, that the anti-aging market is growing at breakneck speed, and that more and more of us are taking preemptive strikes before we even celebrate our twenty-fifth birthdays, treating nonexistent lines with fancy creams—even getting the Stepford Freeze to stop facial expressions in their tracks.[21]

There are new miracle ingredients all the time. There are peptides and antioxidants, gold flakes, and the magical berries from deep in the Amazon. Whether they work or not, most of these anti-aging topicals are nontoxic. Hurray for that. The catch is those miracle ingredients are usually delivered up in lotions packed with other questionable ingredients, and it's hard to know how much of the active ingredient is present in the bottle. To help you pick a good one, we've put together a list of different kinds that are either proven, showing signs of promise, or not worth your time and money at all.

## ANTIOXIDANTS

If you've ever read a woman's magazine, you've heard of the term "free-radical damage." But unless you've always been a biology enthusiast or went on to develop an illustrious career in the field, you might not know what that means. We didn't. In terms of how it ages the skin, here's a simplified explanation:

Normal everyday metabolic function causes the release of "free-radical" molecules. While at certain levels the body can cope with them easily, when produced in excess, these electron-missing rogues can cause damage to other cell structures. There are many contributing factors to the production levels of free radicals, and while they cause us to age, aging itself means our bodies get less good at processing them.[22] How's that for a double-edged sword? Major, major contributors to this sad process are UV rays. Enter antioxidants stage left to combat the free radicals.

While we will look later at the crucial role of antioxidants in our diet, in this chapter we will limit the scope to those that function topically.

**Vitamin C** is pretty much a topical antioxidant rock star, shown to do a number of wonderful things for our skin. It has been reported to help speed wound healing and protect against ultraviolet damage, as well as to increase collagen production and skin density.[23] Other claims to fame include inflammation reduction and an evening effect on skin discoloration. The trick of course is in the delivery; for it to be useful, you need to get enough, and it needs to be stable.[24] Vitamin C oxidizes very easily and when it does, not only does it become useless, it can actually contribute to damage.[25] Some good stabilized C derivatives to look for include L-ascorbic acid, magnesium ascorbyl phosphate, and ascorbyl palmitate. A quick aside: while taking vitamin C is a good idea for other reasons, ingesting the stuff doesn't increase collagen production. [26] It does, however, fend off free-radical damage.

**Vitamin E** is another worthwhile ingredient in anti-aging concoctions. It protects against oxidative damage and UV rays, is a potent antioxidant and can work in tandem with vitamin C when both are stable.[27] Contrary to many a mother, application of E directly on a wound doesn't seem to promote healing,[28] but it does help the skin retain moisture, which is key to its appearance, and also increases the skin's barrier function, which is never a bad thing.[29]

**Pomegranates** and some of their exotic fruity friends have also gotten a lot of airtime. While data on topical applications appear to be inconclusive at this point, there are signs of real promise in the anti-inflammation, wrinkle-fighting department.[30] **Green tea**, an internal antioxidant A-lister, is also emerging with great topical potential (in the form of its ECGG extract) for combating a variety of damaging factors to skin.[31] Some other big antioxidant winners we've read promising things about are **alpha-lipoic acid**,[32] and **coenzyme $Q_{10}$**

$(CoQ_{10})$—which is packed into many wrinkle creams from high-end to drugstore brands, as well as some naturals.[33]

## Vitamin A

Vitamin A has pretty much been crowned queen of the prom when it comes to fighting wrinkles—and she's no slouch at fighting acne, either. But there's more to this antioxidant than meets the eye. Celebrity dermatologist Leslie Baumann told us that while all antioxidants help in the prevention of aging, "only retinoids get rid of wrinkles you already have." Sounds great, but what are retinoids exactly?

Retinoids are compounds derived from retinoic acid, which is a form of vitamin A—tretinoin is the type of retinoid used in popular prescription topicals like Retin-A and Renova. But is it an antioxidant or a peel? In this prescription form it's kind of both: "It increases exfoliation, but it has many more benefits that peels do not have. It increases collagen production and helps keep the collagen-producing genes turned on," Baumann told us.

So what's the catch? For starters, retinoic acid made it onto California's Proposition 65 list for human toxicity, including: "carcinogenicity, reproductive and developmental toxicity, neurotoxicity, and acute toxicity."[34] Second, most tretinoin formulas on the market featured other unfavorables, most notably BHA and BHT (other suspected carcinogens). Tretinoin is also just harsh, sometimes seriously irritating skin, and always making it more susceptible to the sun.[35]

The thing is, tretinoin works—so if it's not the first thing you take off your shelf, we are okay with that. If you're going to take a measured risk, better to do so with a product that's actually delivering some results. Of the ones we looked at, Tazorac cream (not the gel) seemed to be the cleanest—and back before this whole book experiment began, Siobhan was a fan of it. Just be extra careful about the sun, and make sure all of your other products are gentle and clean because your skin will be particularly sensitive while you use these.

Naturally occurring vitamin A also still has wonderful properties, if not the same level of visible effectiveness as its cell-communicating acid analog tretinoin. Holistic skin care specialist Evan Healy told us that certain plant oils, like rosehip seed oil, feature it in abundance: "Research on rosehip seed oil shows that consistent, daily use over a period of four to six months will positively affect cell mitosis, helping to reinforce the supportive scaffolding nature of the skin (collagen production) while also beginning to minimize the appearance of fine lines and wrinkles." Vitamin A is toxic in large amounts, too, though. Do some reading before you buy, and do not take the more-is-better approach.

## DMAE

We're not holding our breath that DMAE is really the facelift in a bottle the world's been waiting for. It is popular in so-called cosmeceuticals, as well as in the fake-natural and real natural markets—but don't let that trick you. Aside from the fact that its benefits have yet to be really proven, the existing good evidence is matched by bad. Take one study in which researchers observed an initial positive cell-protecting response to DMAE, only to discover not long after that it was slowing cell growth, possibly halting it.[36] Another one said this miracle topical can cause "cell death" and that said damage might be the very thing that makes skin appear fuller.[37] It is also considered toxic when inhaled, swallowed, and, surprise, absorbed through the skin.[38] Until more is known, we're not letting it anywhere near our cells.

## Proteins and Other Chains

Peptides are a highly controversial category. The popular palmitoyl pentapeptide (also known by its commercial name Matrixyl) and its wordy relative palmitoyl pentapeptide palmitoyl-lysine-threonine-threonine-lysine-serine (pal-KTTKS), are said to signal collagen production and reduce appearance of wrinkles. The main study we found to support this was based on self-assessments by subjects and was conducted by Procter & Gamble—it owns Oil of Olay, which uses the ingredients in its Regenerist line.[39] There are other claims out there about peptides: some say they can act in a similar way to Botox, blocking transmission signals between nerves, while others say they can help transmit beneficial minerals like copper to the skin.[40]

The real thing about peptides, though, is this: whether or not some controlled study supports any of these claims, we don't buy that companies have figured out a delivery system for them that works. That's because peptides are very unstable; they're water soluble but also can break down in water (that stumped us, too), they don't penetrate skin, and if they did, they'd likely be broken down by the skin's enzymes—so whether they survive in a product, let alone long enough on our faces, has been called into question.[41] What *is* conclusive is that their presence in creams tends to send prices through the roof—believe the hype at your own financial peril.

Some other "ides" that have a bit more scientific muscle behind them are niacinamide (which is vitamin $B_3$) and ceramide. Topical $B_3$ has been shown to reduce appearance of wrinkles, sallowness, and discoloration of skin.[42] Ceramide, meanwhile, is what's called a skin-identical ingredient—it occurs naturally in our skin, helping it look nice, and the topicals are theoretically just like the stuff we produce ourselves. Since we lose ceramide with time and damage, adding it topically in a face cream can be a good idea. The same goes for hyaluronic acid, which is also a natural part of our skin matrix. While topical application will not replace it at a deeper level, it functions as a great humectant, capable of holding a thousand times its weight in water.[43] Other friendly "acids" are linoleic and linolenic—fatty acids found in certain vegetable oils and believed to help reduce inflammation and increase water retention when applied topically (with some other added benefits when consumed).[44]

Not all of these ingredients have made their way into the clean market yet, though many have and others can be bought separately and added to your fave products or home recipes.

A quick warning before we conclude this section: growth factors are creepy. They're being touted as the answer to everything from wrinkles to thicker eyelashes, but we think it's too early to use them, as the risks outweigh the benefits. For instance, epidermal growth factor, which is part of the human growth factor (HGF) family, may cause cell proliferation—great if it's the cells that plump up your skin and terrible when it's cancer.[45] HGFs are confusing, and they're hormones, and the possible dangers associated with long-term topical applica-

tion—let alone how they interact with the rest of our bodies—
are not yet known. It certainly wouldn't be the first time that
the cosmetics industry jumps the gun on using an ingredient
that can cause serious harm.

## Botox, Fillers, and Other Injectibles

This is a slight digression, considering that the FDA *does* "regulate" injectables (since they're drugs). But because most of you
aren't trolling the FDA website with the same enthusiasm as
us, we'll give you a quick rundown. Botox, approved for cosmetic use back in 1989, is the patented name of a product made
of botulinum toxin. Considered to be the most toxic substance
known to humankind, it got its name from the Latin word for
sausage (you can't make this stuff up) because it showed up as
a poison in mishandled meats, causing what became known as
botulism—a rare and paralyzing illness that can lead to respiratory failure.[46] Eventually, it was discovered that using tiny
amounts of the stuff could inhibit localized muscle movement,
which led first to its medical role—treating overactive muscles.
Then, that opened the door to its cosmetic application. Today it
is the most popular anti-aging procedure.

In 2009 the FDA gave Botox the black-box warning—the
agency's most severe safety action, reserved for drugs with
possibly life-threatening effects.[47] Several deaths have been reported in association with Botox, as well as other health issues
as a result of the drug's ability to spread into the body, away
from its injection site. In its press release, however, the FDA
specified that these adverse effects were not associated with
Botox's cosmetic use, but rather with experimental medical

uses that were yet to be approved by the FDA.[48] Fair enough, but not good enough for us.

Facial fillers have also come under some heat. In 2008 the FDA reported that nearly one thousand patients had suffered serious reactions in the previous five years. Some of these included disfigurement, lip and eye paralysis, vision complications, and severe allergic reactions.[49] There is also currently no long-term safety data available on these procedures.[50] But if that doesn't deter you, perhaps this will: on its website, the FDA lists "death of skin" among the risks of using fillers, a possible consequence of accidentally injecting and blocking a blood vessel.[51]

We'll still give these procedures credit where credit is due: they produce visible results (unlike so many of the cosmetics that we put our faith and life savings into). But we find the increasingly breezy attitude people have about this stuff worrisome, in part due to risks, but also because of what we will liken to the ol' gateway-drug theory. When it comes to drugs, we think it's a bullshit postulation, but we kind of do think it applies here. So many women start these procedures with the intention of doing just a little bit, but they lose sight along the way and end up looking like Daffy Duck. (And this doesn't even take into account the potential health dangers.) A friend of ours tried the tiniest injection in her barely noticeable brow furrow; consequently, her forehead, which glistened with that telltale Botox shine, began to fold in weird, unnatural places—lumping in the middle—when she so much as raised her eyebrows.

For those of us who don't look like supermodels, a good part of our physical beauty comes through our facial expressions— the way we look when we smile, crinkle our noses in delight, even the sadness we're able to convey in empathy or in an authentic expression of pain (which also happens to be the same face we make during orgasm). Sure, we all have the desire to preserve our youth—and we may be singing a different tune in twenty years, but for now, we're just not sure where these procedures fit in with aging gracefully.

## Acupuncture Facelifts and Other Alternative Anti-Agers

Just like the mainstream, the green market is also capitalizing on our youth fixation; things like acupuncture and massage "facelifts" as well as facial yoga exercises that promise to keep skin taut are gaining traction among women wary of the chemicals and treatments we've been talking about. As is usually the case with alternative approaches, there's little scientific data to support their claims. While we feel that acupuncture can do pretty magical things, it seems a little far-fetched that the tiny needles could stimulate collagen production (as some claim). On the other hand, that acupuncture could relieve stress and muscle tension in the face seems logical enough, and some women swear they see positive changes: decreased puffiness, brighter complexions, softened lines.[52]

Using massage as a facial technique is certainly nothing new, and while it won't produce facelift-style results, it will increase circulation and aid in lymphatic drainage—not to mention that it just feels great. Finding a good, clean skin care specialist is a fine idea as long as you can afford it and keep your expectations in check. If you can't, don't worry: facial massage is something you can easily do at home when applying your moisturizer (see "The Big Picture" on page 122). Also the book *The Yoga Face* covers some of the facial gymnastics that people swear by.[53]

## THE BIG PICTURE
### A Holistic Expert's Advice on Skin Care

Back before many of us were even picking our noses, let alone thinking about parabens, Evan Healy, now in her fifties, was immersed in the world of natural skin care. What began in the 1980s as a buying job for San Diego's most popular health food store eventually became a new career path for Healy. "I became instantly fascinated, and within a year I decided to get my esthetician's license," she says. "By 1988 I'd begun a private practice in holistic skin care."

By sharing a clinic space with other alternative practitioners, Healy took on a multidisciplinary approach to skin. She began "going sort of rogue," and discovered that sometimes deviating from conventional wisdom revealed "the body's own natural wisdom."

According to Healy, around the time women began to rely more and more on harsh skin treatments—such as acid peels and dermal abrasion—she saw what she calls "schizophrenic skin." "It was across all age lines," she says. "Skin was flaky and dehydrated with broken capillaries, yet also very oily. When I say dehydrated, I don't mean that these women weren't drinking enough water, because they were drinking a ton. And when I say oily, I don't mean just your typical T-zone oil. What was happening was they had so disrupted their skin's natural ability to hold its own moisture, because they were basically dissolving their epidermal layer. The skin was very thin—you can't just destroy a part of this very complex organ and then expect it to do what it's supposed to do."

It probably goes without saying that we like her approach or we wouldn't have turned to her for advice on some of skin's peskiest issues. While some of this may run counter to what you've been taught about skin, there's an inherent logic to what she has to say: "I didn't invent this; I just went back to nature." All righty, then. Let's hear her out.

### Healy on Acne and Basic Skin Maintenance

My general take on acne is that this is the picture of a very sensitive skin type. We should not be aggressive with it. There's some infection and some inflammation, so it also has to be treated from the inside out. If you just treat the acne, it's like shooting the messenger. Skin is an incredible diagnostic organ, so you may have to address food, stress, hormones, elimination.

That said, topically I recommend a very simple formula, and this goes for most things. I think clay is the unsung hero for acne: clay is a living mineral, it's one of the oldest healing materials on earth, and it's present everywhere. It can be really rich in silicon, calcium, iron, magnesium—all of these minerals are strengthening for the skin. Clay has this drawing capacity, so it pulls out dirt and infection as well as excess oil. In ways, it works like an alphahydroxy acid without destroying the epidermal layer, and it helps resolve the infected follicle.

Now cystic acne is a different animal. A regular pimple is very surface, in the epidermal layer, but a cyst is much deeper and just touching it at all can really aggravate it. The one thing you can do when you feel one coming on is to ice it—not so much as to aggravate it more, though, but on and off. Do not touch them or try to lance them.

Whenever I had clients with cystic acne I would see them in conjunction with another healthcare specialist of their choice—an acupuncturist, a doctor, or nutritionist.

### Healy on Rosacea

I have a theory about rosacea. You know, back in the early '90s, I rarely had questions about rosacea, and I rarely saw it. Now I would hazard to say—and maybe I'm exaggerating slightly to make a point—that something like 75 percent of people I talk to preface their questions about skin by saying "I have rosacea." I'm not a doctor, but I think that part of the problem is this "burn model" that is at the core of skin care today. What I'm seeing is this skin that is thinned and reddened, desperately dry—but again it's confused because it's also very oily, too, and there's often the presence of acne with rosacea. Another thing about rosacea that's unlike acne: you can't get rid of it. So you really need to stay attentive to the lifestyle recommendations: avoiding things that create more heat in the body like hot yoga, wine, coffee, stuffy rooms, and so on.

### Healy on Aging

What is all this nonsense about anti-aging? We have this white-knuckled grasp on youth—you know, I want to glow with health, but I don't want my face to be embalmed. Everything I've said about regulating the skin and restoring its ability to self heal is all about preservation—these natural substances help skin to regenerate at a cellular level. When you treat the skin with healthy oils and waters, you get a skin that is more plumped out. These are your best friends when it comes to so-called anti-aging.

## THE FACE GUIDE

FACE

### Soaps and Cleansers

#### Whole Foods Market Triple-Milled Organic Soap

We love this cheap, plant-based bar soap. It's not harsh, it cleans effectively, and you can stock up, thanks to the low price tag. Best of all? It's capped out at around four ingredients, all skin-friendly.

### Ren Mayblossom and Blue Cypress Balancing Facial Cleansing Gel

This U.K. line has a cult following in the United States, and we're card carrying members of the club. We love these sulfate-free gel cleansers—they're more heavy duty than most milks, but don't strip the skin.

### Evan Healy Blue Lavender Cleansing Milk

This is plant-based, oil-and-water mixing at its best. This gentle cleanser was strong enough to dissolve our mascara and foundation, while hydrating the skin, and leaving it nice and soft, even in cool (dry) winter months. We recommend this for all skin types—including those prone to breakouts and rosacea.

### Patyka Organic Face Cleansing Milk and Foaming Face Wash

Light on ingredients (in a good way), these affordable and fair-trade cleansing milk products left our skin clean and makeup-free—but not too clean (also in a good way).

## Moisturizers, Anti-Agers, and Serums

### John Masters Vitamin C Anti-Aging Serum

This wonderful product starts with aloe at the top, followed by some good oils, and then a stable vitamin C. While this one is not food-grade organic (some of Masters's products do go so far), we know that he makes every effort to use top-quality organic ingredients wherever he can.

FACE

*Jurlique Purely Age-Defying Serum*

This is an incredible night serum. You still need to moisturize, but the super-concentrated skin-friendly ingredients pack a punch. It also contains licorice extracts that supposedly help fade uneven sunspots and other discolorations.

*Evan Healy Rosehip Seed Oil*

We love this light oil, which contains naturally occurring vitamin A. (Go back to page 116 and read what Healy has to say about it.) Combine it with a hydrosol for ultimate benefits, and store it somewhere dark—vitamin A is light sensitive. We also can't get enough of the hydrating **Sea Algae Serum**, which we apply right after.

*Dr. Andrew Weil for Origins Plantidote Mega-Mushroom Face Serum*

The ultimate in natural *and* effective, this serum is anti-redness, anti-dryness, and anti-splotch. We saw a noticeable improvement in the dewiness and comfort of our skin after a few weeks.

*Juice Beauty Organic Facial Moisture Concentrate*

Another company that's featuring some USDA certified products in its line (high fives, we know that's not easy)—like this one. Gentle and nourishing, this product also packs an antioxidant punch with its cranberry and grapeseed oil ingredients.

*Ren Hydra-Calm Global Protection Day Cream*

Call us suckers, but we swear that this cream actually feels calm and cooling upon application. It's wonderful for everyday use and full of omegas and calendula. The **Frankincense and Boswellia Serrata Revitalising Repair Cream** for nighttime is no slouch, either.

FACE

## HOW TO WASH YOUR FACE

- Using lukewarm water, wet your face.
- Put a quarter-size amount of clean cleanser in your palm and apply it to your skin with your fingertips, concentrating on areas prone to makeup and congestion.
- The massaging part should take about a minute or two.
- Rinse thoroughly with lukewarm water.
- Pat dry.
- Spray your face with a gentle toner or hydrosol, and don't rub it in. Just let it sit.
- Grab your serum or treatment lotion if you use one, and apply a pea-sized amount to your entire face.
- Wait a minute or two.
- Take the same amount of moisturizer, and apply that all over your face.
- Wait a minute or two.
- Apply sunscreen or makeup, or both, as needed.

*Kahina Giving Beauty 100% Organic Argan Oil (and serum)*
We love Katharine l'Heureux's entire argan-oil based line, but the stand-out here is her pure Moroccan oil, organically grown, harvested by a cooperative of women, and fairly traded. This oil is loaded with antioxidants, absorbs well on damp skin, and is the ultimate multitasker (flyaways, cuticles, face, cuts, elbows, etc.).

*Single Ingredient (Edible and Affordable) Superstars*
If we've said it once, we've said it a thousand times: simplest

FACE

can be best. If you're on a budget, or are just game, we really encourage you to hit the health food store and buy pure ingredients such as **aloe** (the kind they sell to drink is the purest), **coconut, olive,** or **jojoba** oils, and use these as either padding or primary components in your skin care routine. You will get more active benefits this way for far less money, maybe allowing you to splurge on one or two pricier items you love.

### Adding Actives

This is also a great way to save money and still get superstar ingredients. A website called *skinactives.com* specializes in selling all the latest fancy actives at a fraction of the cost. This means you can order them and add them right into your favorite clean cream, or home creation. Careful though: stay away from the too new (and probably unstable) growth factors, peptides, and such. Opt instead for ones from our anti-aging list like **Hyaluronic Acid, Green Tea Extract, Niacinamide,** and **CoEnzyme $Q_{10}$**. Always follow usage instructions carefully.

### Toners

#### John Masters Organics Hydrating Mists

Masters has a pure, USDA organic **Lavender Mist** (which is just lavender flower water) as well as a **Rose and Aloe** one. They're both lovely.

#### Evan Healy Hydrosols

Ok, you get it. We like Healy's products. These were the first ones to really turn us onto hydrosols.

FACE

*Elique Organic Pampered pH*

Elique's hydrosols are also favorites. Get one custom blended for you, or choose one of her well-selected options on offer, depending on your skin type.

## Exfoliants and Peels

*Dr. Hauschka Cleansing Cream*

Less a cream than a gentle scrub, this is a Dr. H mainstay and is one of the only physical scrubs we will even go near. It's gentle enough to use weekly, but can leave skin a little on the slick side, so we prefer to follow up with a gentle cleanser after.

*Juice Beauty Green Apple Peel*

Juice Beauty's whole Green Apple line is devoted to clean AHAs. While we're both too sensitive for those products, many women swear by them. Juice (along with Ren) is also one of the few really clean lines available at Sephora. Don't be fooled by the little green apple, though; this peel is serious stuff. If you're gonna give it a whirl, start with the one for sensitive skin, and do only a few minutes at a time at first (and not the recommended ten).

*Arcona Cranberry Gommage*

If you're going to scrub, go with this. It combines jojoba beads, plant oils, and fruit extracts. The ingredients are pure but powerful.

FACE

## Facial Sunscreen

If you're looking for good mineral makeups that double as broad-spectrum sunscreens, we have our favorites listed in the Chapter 6. We also recommend body sunscreens we like in Chapter 7.

### *John Masters SPF 30 Natural Mineral Sunscreen*
This broad-spectrum sunscreen uses both titanium dioxide and zinc. Compared to many sunscreens we've tried, it really went on light, and while it left a kind of nice glimmer on the skin, it was in no way pasty or white. This is a solid option for all skin tones.

### *Jurlique Purely Age-Defying Day Cream SPF 15*
This works well as a day cream for lighter complexions. It provides great SPF, workhorse anti-agers, and has a nice evening-out effect. It also works well under makeup, but it's not recommended for darker complexions.

### *Soleo Organics*
Clean, affordable, and made with zinc, healthy oils, and green tea extract. We'll say it again in Chapter 7, if you're talking pure sun protection, Soleo is tops. It's probably not what you want to put on your face every day, but if you're going to be out in the sun seriously, keep a tube of this on call.

## Blemish Stuff

### *Organic Apoteke Active Face Hydrating Gel*
This super light gel moisturizer created by a U.K. doctor is per-

FACE

## YOUR FACE AT THE DRUGSTORE

We already mentioned that we like **Burt's Bees** Natural Acne Solutions, but its other face care products are none too shabby, either. We're also fans of the **Jason** line with its heavy emphasis on vitamin C, aloe, cocoa butter, and other good things. Some of the products use parabens, though, and while many use natural fragrance, certain formulations appear to contain the bad stuff. **Alba** and **Yes To** also feature full lines for your face with mostly clean ingredients. **Avalon Organics** has entire lines devoted to actives like vitamin C, $CoQ_{10}$, and soothing lavender. Target even carries beloved brands like **Weleda, Lavera,** and **Juice Beauty**.

fect for oily and irritated skin. It absorbs easily, leaving a matte finish, wears well under makeup, and has in-house clinical trials to back up its blemish-banishing claims. All-star ingredients include neem, fruit extracts, sunflower oil, witch hazel, and coconut oil.

### Jurlique Blemish Cream
Tea tree oil does the hard work here, and the slightly pinkish color makes it suitable for day and night on lighter complexions. It has a drawing effect, bringing zits to the surface more quickly.

### Burt's Bees Natural Acne Solutions
This mostly natural line uses natural salicylic from willow bark as well as calming parsley and antibacterial tea tree, but it's not exactly gentle, so we recommend a light touch.

FACE

*Arcona AM Acne Lotion*
This product features regular acne-busting tea tree oil and the more esoteric totara extract. Totara is a tree that grows in New Zealand, and its extract is shown to be antibacterial.

## Masks

*Jurlique Purifying Mask*
This oil-sopping, zit-calming mask is a favorite of ours (and of Scarlett Johannson's, apparently). It's great to banish breakouts before they come to a head, and have a pleasing, drying effect on surface blemishes, too.

*Elique Organic Skin Food and Evan Healy Clay Masks*
We're devotees of pure clay masks—not the kind you get at the drugstore that strip the skin, but the mineral and nutrient-rich clays from smaller companies. Elique's Conquer clay mask does an awesome job decongesting our pores, without the overly drying effect of some other clays, and Evan Healy's powder clay (you add the water yourself, which means it has no preservatives and doesn't spoil) is unbelievably soft and soothing.

FACE

# 6

## Your Makeup

Perhaps you have noticed we're both kind of evangelists. If we love a new pair of jeans, we think everyone should at least try them on. If we discover Campari, we think everyone should ditch their vodka sodas. This is especially true of beauty products, partly because there's just something about a new bottle of goop that turns us on. And if it gets us excited, we want to share it with the world.

Of course, that's kind of tricky in a beauty book. We're all different. One size does not fit all, and that is especially true of makeup. We understand that women spend years trying to find the right shade of red for their kissers and the silkiest finish for their foundation. We also understand that once you've found something you like, it's a hard sell to get you to switch—especially because of what we're going to tell you next.

### MEET YOUR (NATURAL) MAKEUP

Despite our inclination to promise—not unlike the beauty companies—that you can have it all as you switch to clean makeup, it's not totally true. There are colors that cannot be made naturally; foundations for darker complexions can be hard to find; and since lots of this stuff is available mostly online, color matching can be a pain.

Also, naturals just don't perform the same way. They're not worse (in fact, we think many are better), but they're definitely different. Why? For starters, some of those chemical-laden products are indeed longer-lasting (at a cost, mind you). Not to mention that these companies have had decades to perfect their formulas.

That being said, having dinner with nary a smudge on your lipstick strikes us as totally creepy—up there with tattooed eyebrows. As natural makeup artist Jessa Blades puts it: "We need to rethink what we expect of these products. If you have to reapply, you have to reapply."

The upshot is that even before the advent of modern beauty chemistry, chicks did their faces. So read on. In addition to finding some natural lines we absolutely love, we also learned a few tricks from makeup artists along the way that we will share with you (see page 145). Because as Blades points out, "We do not need a million new makeup lines; what we need is to learn how to apply it properly." Amen, to that.

### Liquid Foundation and Tinted Moisturizer

We're going to come right out and say it: we find most foundation gross. Like skin-crawling, nose-scrunching, get-it-outta-here gross. Why? Just open up your makeup case and check the bottle. The first ingredient is probably water, which immediately means there are going to be loads of synthetic preservatives in

there. Next, you'll find a cocktail of silicones, chemical sunscreens, fragrance, mineral oil, waxes, and those carcinogen-
releasing chemicals we keep talking about. The one quality all
those ingredients share is the fact that none of them are good
for your skin. It's just pore-clogging, skin-dulling crap that
makes you think you need it to look lovely. Nothing pretty
about that.

Healthy skin aside, bad foundation is guilty of more makeup
crimes than dark lip liner. Everyone's seen the lady with the orange face, or the too-thick foundation that cakes into fine lines.
It's just not attractive, mainly because it doesn't look like skin.
Still, we're no strangers to skin problems, so we understand
the role this stuff plays; it can give you the coverage you need
on those days when you want to put a paper bag over your
head and cry.

If you wear foundation twice a year, wear whatever you
want. But if it's your main source of coverage, your moisturizer, and your daily SPF, then this is the first thing in your
makeup kit to replace. If you're choosing a new liquid or
cream-solid foundation, look for ones with a physical sunscreen (zinc or titanium dioxide) and nonirritating oils like jojoba or castor, organic beeswax and natural (but nonirritating)
herbal extracts and vitamins.

A couple of years ago, the stuff on the nontox market kind of
blew, but these days, there are some pretty sophisticated options out there. Best of all, some of them are actually good for
your skin. Celebrity fashion makeup artist Rose-Marie Swift—
who has been dolling up models for *Vogue, Harper's Bazaar,
W,* and many others for years—insists on using only nourishing
ingredients in her line, RMS Beauty. "I use oils with a long shelf
life," she says. "Coconut oil and jojoba oil are great and work

with the skin. Safflower oil and olive oil are cheap. The secret to any good product is the ingredients. I don't even use essential oils because there's a lot of documentation that they cause rashes and irritation."

These days, we really like mixing truly clean mineral makeup with rms's "un" cover-up spread lightly over problem areas, for example. The former is anti-inflammatory, and the latter is moisture-rich, oil-gland-calming deliciousness.

## Concealers

Generally speaking, concealers contain the same ingredients as foundations, only they have less liquid and more pigment. If you have one you love and you apply it at the end of your makeup, on top of a base, then it's not the end of the world if it's not totally clean. But if you're wearing it to hide pimples (which often means broken skin), beware. Broken skin makes for easier penetration and irritation, and this could just compound the problem. You've no doubt seen treatment concealers with tea tree oil (or benzoyl peroxide if it's a conventional zit-zapper). We think these are pricey gimmicks that will irritate your skin and drain your wallet. Most do not contain enough of the active ingredient to make much of a difference, so the chances of it healing while it covers are not high. We also think clean mineral powders can serve as excellent spot coverers because they're easy to layer and don't look cakey if you apply them properly. The other hot things on the market are color-correcting concealers to help neutralize undereye blues and blacks, and zitty reds. Unless you're talking about extreme discoloration, you probably don't need to fork over another couple bills for one of these. Just learning how to apply a good concealer that matches your skin should do the trick.

### Loose and Compact Powders and Minerals

Powders, both mineral and non, make up a huge portion of the market for a few reasons: they're comparatively cheap; can look quite elegant; and can provide excellent coverage without making you look like you're wearing a face full of makeup. They can also be pretty problematic because you're at risk of breathing them in, and also because they're often coated with crap.

Let's focus on minerals for a second. This is the fastest-growing makeup market, which means that it's also packed with fakes that offer the same old garbage with minerals sprinkled in to please some marketing department and boost sales. "The mineral lines are playing games," says Swift. "They coat them with parabens, and some dry out the skin. And the ones that are silky and smooth have silicones in them."

Indeed, the real stuff—which is literally made of pulverized minerals and very little else—can be great, though. Scan ingredient lists and you're bound to see titanium dioxide (which is what makes it opaque and provides SPF), mica (which gives a light-reflecting shimmer), and iron oxides. Some also contain bismuth oxychloride, which can refract light and look pretty, but can also be an irritant and dry out the skin. (Most people who tend to get rashes or break out from mineral makeup are reacting to this stuff. It's nontoxic, though.[1])

In a good-quality product, mineral makeup can create a nice evening effect, where you can still see skin underneath. While we won't cosign claims that you should sleep in them, or that they'll make your rosacea go away, we will allow that they're an awesome decoy for flaws, and that it can make you look good enough to sleep *with*. We're both fans with just one important caveat: you have to pick a truly clean one. Wait, two caveats: you also can't snort the stuff.

Because titanium dioxide tends to create a whitish effect, it has some drawbacks. Generally speaking, it works best on lighter complexions because, as many a beauty guru has pointed out, it can look ashy on darker skin.[2] To counter the pallor, some companies are trying to go with much smaller particles—as in, *nano*, small. Nanos are of concern because their widespread use is relatively new. They're thought to penetrate easily, and there's just a lot we don't know about how they behave in the body. Titanium dioxide nanoparticles, for what it's worth, are thought *not* to penetrate healthy skin.[3] We wouldn't bet our shoe collections that someone won't some day come out and say these nanos are a no-no, though. It's a lung toxicant, which means even applying loose powder with titanium and zinc in it around your nose and mouth requires some caution. If you're concerned or have a baby or small child, go for pressed powder—less floating around in the air that way.

As for nonmineral powders, most are talc-based. Talc, you now know, is verboten. Many also contain bismuth oxychloride, which can contain irritating parabens, aluminum compounds, silicones, and PEG. Cornstarch (sometimes listed as zea mays) is nontoxic and is also used in a lot of face powders and blushes by mainstream brands like Nars and Almay, as well as health-food-store staples like Miessence. It sits nicely on the skin, but acne-prone ladies beware: it can help feed acne-causing bacteria—or so we've been told. If your skin likes any excuse for an eruption, you'll want to avoid any face products that contain it.

## Lipstick

If makeup has a single shining star, it's gotta be lipstick. Not only is it the most popular tool in the kit, nothing changes our faces so quickly and dramatically as that simple stroke of color. And while our mouths are sexual signifiers enough, there is also a trite (but probably true) claim that lips intimate their vulval twins below, and that to paint them is to mimic that nether blush of arousal. No wonder it was reserved for prostitutes during certain more austere periods of history, like Queen Victoria's England.[4]

Cleopatra and her team of makeup innovators were the first ones to use crushed (and impregnated[5]) female cochineals—disgusting little insects that live on cacti—to get the perfect red lip. The little buggers were later rediscovered by the Aztecs, and then stolen by the Spaniards, who would end up holding a monopoly on the potent red dye for some two hundred years.[6] A hugely valuable commodity then and still, cochineal continues to be a popular coloring agent in foods, fabric dyes, and of course, your favorite red lipstick.[7]

Ew-factor aside, the bugs are the least of it. Our lipsticks, which we both absorb and accidentally eat (you know it's true), are often contaminated with lead. Yes, the poisonous neurotoxin. Back in 2007 when the Campaign for Safe Cosmetics tested a batch of thirty-three lipsticks, more than 60 percent of them contained lead.[8] Well, this got international attention, pushing the FDA to do its own study in 2009. Using a new, more sophisticated method for detecting lead, its results proved even more shocking: *all* twenty lipsticks it tested contained lead. While the FDA doesn't set lead limits for cosmetics, it does set them in candy (why any lead would be in candy is beyond us); on average, the lipsticks contained ten times the levels that are in candy.[9] When you consider how often some of us are smearing on the toxic smack, the common defense—that even these amounts are harmless—starts to sound increasingly hollow.

Don't believe us? Here's what Dr. Michael DiBartolomeis from California's Department of Public Health had to say: "If there is lead in any of these cosmetics, then that should get people pretty ticked off. There's no reason for it. Lead should absolutely not be in any of these products." Ah, but they are! And women who wear lipstick during their pregnancy are unknowingly exposing their fetuses to lead. Like mercury in fish, this needs to be taken seriously.

We're not done yet. Popular lipsticks also contain BHA, a controversial fat preservative that's used in food, and is "reasonably anticipated to be a human carcinogen" by government agencies like the EPA and NIEHS.[10] That conclusion doesn't come easy: it means there is enough varied animal data, in this case in rats and hamsters, showing BHA to be cancerous.[11] While some studies have shown BHA and its controversial cousin BHT to have positive antioxidant effects, we feel that these are undone by the potential risks.[12] Lipstick can also contain nano-particles, and of course the regulars: fragrance, parabens, propylene glycol, *et al.*

The upshot is that in this category we really don't need to settle. Some of our favorite brands make lipsticks we love: glossy, shiny, and matte, that feel as good as they look.

## Lip Balms

Remember those rumors of Chapstick addiction? There was always that girl (maybe she was you) manically reapplying it every five minutes. Well, the schoolyard claims might have been true after all: most commercial lip balms that are supposed to moisturize dry lips exacerbate the problem. It's no wonder then that the more you use the chem-stick, the more you feel you need to. (This is starting to be a common theme, no?) Your basic balm is probably a petrochemical base, like white petrolatum, with alcohol high on the ingredients list, some chemical sunscreen, like PABA, fragrance, parabens, etc.

Fear not, though: there are much better and simpler ways to get soft lips. Burt's Bees, for one, makes a great standby. We also love Intelligent Nutrients's.

## Lip Gloss and Plumpers

Sorry to say, your glosses aren't doing you any favors, either. They also usually contain alcohol, and anyone who's had a hangover knows how drying that is, along with some variation of the bad stuff you find in lipstick and balms. Ever paid fifty bucks for a lip plumper that claims to fill your lips with collagen and hyaluronic acid? Well, we have, and while there may be trace amounts of those ingredients in there (not enough to "fill" anything), most of the product is the usual garbage. Good ol' Vaseline would probably pump your lips more—not that we're recommending it, but at least it's proven to lock moisture in. We've also already mentioned that hyaluronic acid is a nice active ingredient and that you can buy it and add it to your clean products for extra kick.

## Mascara

If you poke around online, you can find some pretty horrifying things about mascara. Some of it is merited and partly used as a rallying tool because all women wear the stuff every day. Also, it goes near our eyes. Talking trash about things that go near our eyes (or our babies) is usually a good way to get people's attention. At the same time, do you really want formaldehyde releasers, mercury, SLS, coal tar, petroleum distillates, vinyl, parabens, phthalates, and triethanolamine dripping into your eyeballs?

Us neither, and mascaras often contain all of them at a time. Ask any clean girl and she'll tell you that nothing tested her spirit like the hunt for a mascara that's as good as the dirties. Josie Maran even told us that she wouldn't launch her line until she'd perfected her own paraben-free mascara. (It's great, by the way.)

The so-called natural market is moving so quickly, though, that from the time we started writing this book until now, at least a half dozen new clean or clean*er* mascaras we like have hit the market. In the cleans you might find waxes, mineral pigments, some conditioning oils and extracts, clay, and sometimes alcohol. Purists will tell you the ones with alcohol aren't green. We'll agree that it can be irritating, but in our recommendations in "The Makeup Guide" at the end of this chapter we've found some that *do* contain alcohol but perform well and have not bugged our eyes one bit.

## Eye Shadow and Liner

If you've ever slept in your contacts or had conjunctivitis, you know how sensitive eyes are. Our peepers are incredibly delicate, and yet many of us have suffered through the irritations of liners and shadows in the name of a dramatic look, not giving a second bat to the fact that we're absorbing this crap through ultra-sensitive mucous membranes in our eyes.[13]

The smoky eye wasn't always just about sex appeal, though. Back in ancient Egypt, they thought the dark kohl lining protected against eye ailments as well as the sun's glare. Kohl is still very popular in many parts of the world: some Muslims wear it in imitation of their Prophet, who was believed to sleep in the stuff, and many Indians adorn their babies with it.[14] It's a great look; the only problem is that the stuff used to be lead-based, which isn't all that good for babies (or us). While commercially available kohls no longer contain lead, now they're more like glorified eyeliner. The good news—there's an easy way to "make" your own (see page 147).

Eyeliner is one of our favorite products: a night on the town just doesn't seem complete without it. It's not the dirtiest product on your face, but when you consider that some of us use it *inside* our eyes, it should be nothing short of clean. Your run-of-the-mill black pencil liner probably contains polyethylene, a bonding agent that can be contaminated with super-scary 1,4-dioxane, as well as parabens, mineral oil, and paraffin. Some liquid ones also contain propylene glycol, while a few had crazy shit like DMDM (which releases formaldehyde upon contact with the body) and BHT in them. Not in our eyes, thanks.

Shadows are a whole other story, from aluminum powder to silica (which can have lead contamination), BHT to BHA, to nanos—there's a whole variety of crap in these, whether we're talking about the pretty powder variety or the creamy kind. On the plus side, there are a few new lines out that we love, offering concentrated pigment and lasting color.

### Blush, Bronzer, and Shine

Whether it's too many drinks, not enough sleep or just some bad office lighting, most of us have good reason to reach for a little something to enhance our natural glow. There are powders, there are creams, there are tints, and while they may make us *look* healthier, you know they're probably doing just the opposite.

Blush, which is still called rouge in some circles, was initially more of a creamy, cheek-lip hybrid. We used to be big fans of finger-painting lipstick on our cheeks (lead cheeks!), so it's no wonder that one of our new absolute favorite products is a throwback to that double-dip concept. There's just something so easy about matching your cheek tone to your lips, and using your finger—God's intended makeup brush—to do it. Conventional cream blush though? Keep your fingers out. It's just another super chemy concoction of ingredients contaminated with stuff like lead and 1,4-dioxane, along with about twenty other things that don't belong on your pretty cheeks.

The same goes for the powders, whether we're talking about blush or bronzer. Most of them contain a similar mix of synthetics—silica, polyethelyne, methylparaben, and fragrance. There's no shortage of clean mineral options in this category, though, whether you prefer a loose or pressed blush or bronzer—as we already mentioned earlier, mineral makeup can be a fabulous choice, as long as you're getting the clean ones and following a few basic application rules.

If you love a good cheek stain, like the perennial favorite Benetint, we've got a nearly identical alternative you can make in your kitchen (see page 150).

## Luminizers

Luminizers are kind of a loose subcategory: they're really any product designed to add a little dewy splash to the face, sometimes simply by catching the light. If you've never tried one, do (from our list, of course)—it can be just the right detail to a made-up face in the evening, or so lovely with a nearly nude day look if your skin's on good behavior. Some of the conventional ones look more like lip gloss, while others are shimmery powders; often some shine is built into a blush or bronzer. Obviously, those ones are all full of crap. This was one product, though, that we never had to say goodbye to since we only fell for luminizers when we discovered the incredible clean ones out there. Now we can't live without them.

---

### INSIDER TIPS FROM
### NATURAL MAKEUP ARTIST JESSA BLADES

Jessa Blades spent years learning about makeup—at the Makeup Artistry School in Toronto and at the makeup company M.A.C.—so when she first started hearing that makeup might be a serious occupational hazard, she was a little skeptical. "I would hear there's lead in lipstick," she says, "and then I would hear there isn't, which was a relief because lipstick is really pretty, and I wanted to use it on my clients." Over time, though, she did more and more research, and became outraged at what she discovered.

"As a makeup artist, the back of my hand is my canvas. Women make choices all the time that are bad . . . like smoking or wearing high heels, but we know smoking kills, we know high heels hurt our feet. But with beauty products, we are not told that our lipstick could have neurotoxins in it."

So down the rabbit hole she went, and it's a good thing she did. Now, the *Glamour* magazine eco hero spends her time doing makeup, educating women about safe alternatives, and teaching them how to apply makeup properly. Because she has tried pretty much every brand in the naturals' market—not to mention working with the mainstream for years—she has a better grasp than most on what works. It makes the trial-and-error game a little easier for all of us. So without further ado, here are a few tips we picked up.

### Blades on Foundation

You need it only in the center of your face, gently spread out from there. You do not need foundation on your hairline, or your jaw line, or your neck. Right now, I really like RMS concealer and tinted moisturizers from Dr. Hauschka.

### Blades on Bronzer

I am one of those people who thinks everyone looks good in a bronzer. You can use a tiny bit mixed into your primer or foundation. It evens you out and gives an overall healthy glow.

### Blades on Your Favorite Red Lipstick

You do not need to change the fancy red lipstick that you wear every six months. We're talking about daily use and its buildup. Keep your lipstick.

*Blades on Concealing Zits*

Use the tiniest amount of concealer you can with a hard brush. Let it sink in for a minute, very lightly buff it, top it with powder and then leave it alone. Oilier skin needs to be touched up more often.

*Blades on Mascara*

First of all, curl your lashes. Now, I don't usually think eyelash primers work, but Jane Iredale has a great one. You can build on it and use less mascara. One of my favorite mascaras is Couleur Caramel, which is like the Dior Show of naturals.

*Blades on Your Makeup Brushes*

I cannot stress this enough. You have to wash them regularly. In a perfect world, you do this every week or every other week.

---

# MAKE YOUR OWN MAKEUP

We love the *idea* of making our own cosmetics. It's kind of like the fantasy we have about one day growing all of our own food, making jams, pickling things, and only riding a bike. There are a few books and websites out there that can teach you how to make a lot of your own natural makeup. We have pored over them excitedly, full of big intentions to spend a Saturday turning our kitchens into cosmetics labs. But unless you're already the jam girl (bless your heart, can we be friends?) our sense is that most of us have other stuff to do.

So, what we're going to do here is beyond basic. Let's think of it as a survival guide, in the event that a tornado ripped

## HOW TO PROPERLY WASH YOUR MAKEUP BRUSHES

- By now, we're going to assume every shampoo in your bathroom is squeaky clean. Grab any one that you like from the side of the tub, and squeeze a dime size into the palm of your hand.
- Wet the soap and then gently coat each brush with suds.
- Using circular strokes, loosen up the crud on the bristles, being careful not to smoosh them flat into your palm. This can ruin your brushes and loosen the glue that keeps the bristles attached to the wand.
- Next, pinch out the soapy water from the base to the tip until the water runs clear.
- When all your brushes are washed, grab your conditioner (seriously) and stroke each brush through a tiny dab in your palm, gently coating the bristles.
- Rinse well, again pinching the water from base to tip, until they don't feel slick anymore. This will extend the life of your brushes, and if your conditioner isn't giving you acne, it won't mess up your face, either. (If it *is*, for crying out loud, get a new one.)
- To dry them, lay them flat on the edge of your sink or counter. Do this at night. By morning, you have bacteria- and grime- and oil- and makeup-free brushes.
- Repeat biweekly. Your face will thank you.

through your town and destroyed all the CVS's. Or say you're running super late for a hot date—bam, your eyeliner breaks, and the last time you owned a pencil sharpener was in grade school. Or maybe you're just really, really trying to save cash (hey, we're with you). Well, this little DIY makeup guide could come in handy. The rules are simple: only one or two ingredients required per "product" and minimal to no preparation.

## Eyeliner

If you've ever had food poisoning or just really bad gas, you may be familiar with a miraculous little remedy known as activated charcoal. We keep capsules of this stuff around and one day had the genius idea of opening one up. There it was: perfect, pure black powder. This is an amazing eye kohl, smudge, or sleek black liner, depending on what brush you use. We like the small, flat, and stiff type because it gives you more control. If you want a true liquid line, just blend in a tiny bit of your favorite oil and you're good to go. Don't have activated charcoal? Grab an almond, put it on a spoon that you don't mind ruining, and heat it like crack. Ta-da: black powder.

## Mascara

Same as above, except this time, mix in a little bit of oil and/or a touch of aloe vera gel with your powder and use an old mascara wand to apply. We're not going to say that this is the miracle mascara, but it does the trick in a pinch.

## Brows

If you're lucky enough to have real black eyebrows, do the same as mascara; just add more aloe so that they don't look painted on. Otherwise just aloe vera and an old mascara wand (cleaned off) is a great way to keep unruly eyebrows in place.

## Shadow

If pure black shadow is not your vibe, one of our friends recommends using spirulina powder. For those who don't know, spirulina is a kind of blue-green algae. We've never been a big fan of colored eye shadows on ourselves, but we admire them on others. While spirulina might sound super hippie-weird, it's already used in cosmetics for both its beautiful color and its incredible nutritional properties. So there.

## Lips and Cheeks

We have one word and one word only: beets! This is nature's Benetint. There are a few ways to do it, but this is what we like best: cut a small piece of raw beet and use the juicy side to apply directly to lips and cheeks. It's that easy. There are a few reasons why this is so awesome: (1) beets are super healthy, filled with antioxidants and known to be great for skin when consumed; (2) the stain lasts, which, if you've ever cooked with beets, you know is true; (3) because this is translucent (though very bright), it really works on any complexion; and (4) whole beets last forever in the fridge, so you can just keep cutting small pieces off the same one.

However, if you feel weird about carrying a small piece of beet wrapped in foil around in your purse, we have some suggestions. Go to your local juice bar and order pure beet juice.

Fill a small dropper or one of those little brown essential oil bottles with some of the juice, and carry it with you. For a less intense color, mix the beet juice with some of your favorite oil and use it more like a gloss-slash-luminizer: such a pretty pink shine. Just the juice will go bad faster, though, so if you're going to do this, make weekly itty-bitty batches and keep it in the fridge when you're home.

We've also heard that it's super easy to make an actual lip gloss using beets, beeswax and oil, but that broke our two ingredient rule and the idea of heating up wax (and having to clean it) made us tired. We have every intention of trying it someday, of course, and encourage you to as well.

## THE MAKEUP GUIDE

*Foundations, Tinted Moisturizers, and Concealers*

*Lavera Tinted Moisturizer and Lavera Makeup Fluid*
Both of these award-winning favorites offer up nice, even coverage. While the moisturizer is slightly more translucent, it also packs the hydrating power of hyaluronic acid. Just depends what you're after.

*Nvey Eco Organic Liquid Foundation*
We have to distinguish here between Nvey's cream foundation, which we don't adore, and the liquid foundation, which may be one of the best we've ever tried. We're talking flawless finish

MAKEUP

meets the super-soothing ingredients of cucumber and chamomile.

### RMS Beauty "un" cover-up

We're basically obsessed with this stuff. It's the purest makeup line out there, created by none other than the legendary makeup artist Rose-Marie Swift. We basically love her whole line, and we're not alone—Gisele and Karolina do too. The absence of silicones means no fingerprints and easy blending; the oils make it nourishing for the skin and give the complexion a dewy, youthful appearance. We could go on. Stock up.

### Jane Iredale Dream Tint Moisturizer

This stuff is lovely. It comes out thick, and you don't need much—rub it around in your hands and sweep it over your cheeks and forehead for a smoothing look without too much coverage (SPF included).

### W3LL People Narcissist Mineral Cream Foundation

This stuff is dewy, goes on like a dream, and comes in a tube for easy portability and application on the go. Great as a base or primer, or on its own.

## Loose and Pressed Mineral Powders

### Laura Mercier Mineral Powder

This is the best mineral powder we've tried. From a mainstream makeup line, this zinc oxide–packed powder foundation contains only a handful of ingredients, exacted our hard-to-match skin colors, and lasted for hours of subtle but

MAKEUP

great coverage. Any makeup that garners multiple "your skin looks great" comments is good enough for us.

### Bare Escentuals bareMinerals SPF 15 Foundation

The purity and simplicity of the foundation is what appeals to us most, and coverage is impressive. Use it as an all-over base or with a concealer brush over imperfections. The only catch is that it contains bismuth oxychloride, which breaks some people out.

### Jane Iredale Amazing Base and Pure Pressed Minerals

The loose powder is a close match to Bare, but without the bismuth. The coverage is more on the medium side (skin definitely peeks through), which makes for a better summer look. The compact, meanwhile, is more appealing for its portability and mirror.

### Alima Pure

Alima minerals are affordable and cover the largest range of complexions for base foundation—from cool to warm to neutral, palest pales to richer browns. You can order samples from them for a buck fifty, which is great for color-matching to your skin. They also have extremely helpful customer service.

## Mascara

### Couleur Caramel Mascara

This favorite among the non-tox crowd gives a really full lash and does not flake. CC also lets you choose between two different brushes: one for length and one for thickness. We do

MAKEUP

both on occasion—one coat of length, wait, then one coat of thick.

### Dr. Hauschka Volume Mascara

This is a solid, everyday mascara. It won't give you red-carpet eyes (or bedroom ones, for that matter), but it doesn't run, goes on nice and dark, and is completely harmless. It even contains neem oil, which is thought to be good for hair.

### Tarte Lash Hugger

Not the cleanest of the bunch, but this paraben- and petro-chemical-free mascara is a great alternative to the mainstreams. It's widely available, goes on nice and thick, and has one of the better application brushes in the group.

### Josie Maran Mascara

Again, maybe not for diehard purists, but this mascara in black is a true winner for our money. It's one of our favorites because it adds thickness, lasts all day, and won't run down your face unless you wear it to the gym (or have a cry).

### Jane Iredale PureLash Mascara

This is a more natural lash, but can also be built upon since it does not clump. Iredale also does the **Longest Lash Thickening & Lengthening Mascara** if you're going for more intensity. Don't forget the **Extender & Conditioner** that was recommended by Jessa Blades as a primer.

## Lips

### RMS Beauty Lip2Cheek
This is another one of our favorite discoveries. These cute little pots of creamy color are food-grade organic and filled with some of our most trusted skin care ingredients. Best applied with a finger, they look amazing on lips *and* cheeks.

### All the Better to Kiss You With Lip Balm
These darling little antique-looking cases are cheap, amazingly hydrating and are certified USDA organic—which is particularly appealing since we all know you can't avoid accidentally eating your lip balm.

### Couleur Caramel Lipstick
These taste good, wear long, and come in richly pigmented colors. You can get pearlescent ones or matte and, rest assured that unlike the crushed-bug lipsticks that currently occupy your kit, these are loaded with good-for-you ingredients. We love their True Red and Old Rose.

### Josie Maran Lipstick
This product has a really lovely, smooth feel on the lips and comes in a variety of earth-toned pinks, with one or two deeper shades. It's a more subtle look—definitely great for everyday wear.

### Burt's Bees Balms and Lip Shimmer
Burt's offers up a wide variety of basic lip balms, but we were surprised at how much we liked their color line, too—they

MAKEUP

really cover those pinky-wine-mauvey-browns in all of their yummy shades (you know, raisin, rhubard, merlot . . . ).

### Juice Organic Lip Moisturizer

If you like a shiny, wet lip, then Juice Organics makes the perfect gloss for you. It looks great alone or blended with a color to turn any lipstick into a sheerer gloss, with lots of healthy oils to lock moisture into lips.

### Intelligent Nutrients Lipbalm

This is hands down the most nourishing, nonaddictive, delicious-smelling, and effective lip moisturizer we've ever used. Put it on before bed, over lip stains, or lay it on thick for a shimmery look.

### W3LL People Nudist Lip Shine

Created by a dermatologist/makeup artist/hippie trio, this entire line is packed with skin-friendly ingredients and comes in richly pigmented palettes. The Nudist lip balms are amazing, go on thick, stay put, and one of the shades reminds us of a Clinique best-seller: Black Honey Almost Lipstick.

### W3LL People Universalist Multistick

These are go-anywhere sticks of insanely concentrated pigment that you can work into the skin for a gentle flush, or build to levels of intensity that are hard to find in naturals. The red is the reddest natural we've found and can look insanely dramatic (in the best way). We like the pinks and reds best.

MAKEUP

## Eyeliners/Shadows

### Jane Iredale Eyeliner Pencil

This is your standard black (or brown, or blue, or grey, or taupe) pencil liner. Every girl needs one of these, and it's a no-compromise transition.

### Jane Iredale Liquid Eyeliner

Yes, Jane again. We really get into the black, but for more adventurous types this also comes in silver, gold, brown, copper, and pinot noir. Suggestions by eye color are made on its website.

### Suki Triple Cream Eye Definer

Other things we love: multipurpose products that work. This creamy number can go on lids and brows, or be used as a liner. Great texture and a unique, if slightly limited, color selection.

### Alima Pure Luminous Shimmer Eyeshadows

If more color and pizzazz is what you're after, you must check out this incredible selection. We're talking like fifty amazing colors here, and you can order sample sizes for just a buck off the website. Smart.

### Josie Maran Eye Shadow

One of the things we love most about Josie's line is, honestly, the packaging and feel of the products. Esthetics are important with makeup, and this a great gateway line for girls who want to try natural without being crunchola. Her shadows are particularly standout. Great colors, too.

MAKEUP

---

## YOUR MAKEUP AT THE DRUGSTORE

We already mentioned how delighted we were to discover **Physician's Formula Organic Wear** at Target, and it appears to be popping up in some drugstores as well. For the most part, though, you're not going to find a whole lot of clean makeup at your local pharmacy. The **Almay Pure Blends** line, however, is cleaner and becoming widely available, as are the **Burt's Bees** balms and shimmers we love so much. Target, championing again, appears to carry a lot of **Lavera**'s makeup line, including liners, mascara, concealers, and so on.

---

## Bronzers and Luminizers

### RMS Beauty Living Luminizer

This stuff gives you that just-woke-up-from-a-nap-had-sex-and-then-took-a-bath look. It works amazingly well under concealer to camouflage undereye shadows, on cheekbones, on your middle-upper lip to accentuate your pout, or dabbed on your eyelids right above your iris, to perk up your entire face in the most unfussy way. Every girl should own it. (We promise we're not on her payroll.)

### Josie Maran Bronzing Argan Oil

We're obsessed with this stuff. We love argan oil, period, but we're especially fond of Josie's tinted oil for that summer sunkissed look. It's dewy but it absorbs well. You can use it on

MAKEUP

your cheekbones and brow bones as a luminizer, or dab a little in your palms and smooth over your whole face or arms for an allover glow.

*Physicians Formula Organic Wear 2-in-1 Bronzer and Blush*
This brand is an affordable and delightfully good bronzer we found at Target. More St. Tropez than Miami (sorry, Florida), it's subtle, non-orangey, and works year-round. We like the neutral blush it comes with, too, though each can be bought separately in an array of shades.

## Blush

*Vapour Organic Beauty Aura Blush*
Torch is their brightest fuchsia, and it wears amazingly well on cheeks and lips, on a wide range of complexions. It's pure pigment, goes on smooth, and can be layered for a more dramatic nighttime look. And don't worry—it looks bolder in the tube than it does on your skin.

*Dr. Hauschka Rouge*
This is a basic powder blush that works great for every day. There's a universality to the pinks and browns—we can't imagine a complexion they wouldn't work on—and it lasts longer than most of the cream blushes out there.

*Alima Blushes*
These come in mattes and shimmers in an astounding range of colors, from I-just-worked-out flushes to more dramatic shades

MAKEUP

for night. They're sold in little pots of loose powder, so they are probably better for at-home application with a brush, but with a little moisturizer on your finger, you could dip in and smear it on for more of a stain on the go.

MAKEUP

# 7

## Your Body

Science tells us skin is our biggest organ, that it's a living, breathing thing—there to protect us and keep our innards from falling out. Then, in the same breath, it tells us we can put whatever we want on it, as long as the bottle says "for external use only." So we take heed and don't drink our body lotion. But we know now what does drink it: our skin. All the way into our bloodstreams.

In this chapter we're going to familiarize you with how certain parts of our body functions. It's fascinating stuff, and it helps you understand why some ingredients work better than others. We'll look at the main ones in lotions, self-tanners, deodorant, hair-removers, cellulite creams, and stretch mark lotions, and help you find effective replacements for all of them. Promise.

### MEET YOUR BODY

You'll hear it a lot: skin is made up of five layers, and it is our first line of defense—there to keep the bad stuff out of the rest of you. But girls, just because it keeps out the rain does not it a rubber coat make. Absorption of contaminants in water has been grossly underestimated. While we sit around worrying if our water bottles are okay to drink out of, an average of 64 percent of that danger comes from what we're taking in through our skin, not just our mouths.[1] So buy a showerhead filter—they're widely available, and they come cheap. There. Now that's one less thing you have to worry about.

Meanwhile, you probably take your whole body through a ritual of cleansing, hydrating, scrubbing, deodorizing, and hair removal, but we're going to guess that by comparison you're just not as careful with it as you are your face. We're going to suggest you get careful, though, because you're covering twenty or so square feet of you with product. The products you use every day, and over a large area of your body, are the ones that need the most attention. On the bright side, they're also some of the easiest to replace in your routine: (1) because the body-care market is big, so there are more options, and (2) because most of us are less attached to our shaving cream than we are to our favorite lipsticks, you'll probably be less finicky about making changes. Read on for some great recommendations, but before that, of course, there is some insight into the stuff we've all been covering ourselves in for way too long.

## Body Cleansers: Washes, Soaps, and Scrubs

Like shampoo and face wash, body cleansers serve the pretty straightforward purpose of washing away dirt, grime, and dead skin cells. So many, though, using harsh cleansers to get the job done, also strip away beneficial natural oils in the process, making skin dry (necessitating moisturizer), flaky (necessitating harsh exfoliants), and more susceptible to the chemicals packed into these and other products. In their favor, because they are designed with the goal of residue-free rinsing, cleansers are rarely the worst terrorists on the flight.

But let's not be letting them off the hook just yet. You may recall that certain surfactants produce an unlisted carcinogenic byproduct called 1,4-dioxane. Let's do a quick refresher: 1,4-dioxane gets a full ten-out-of-ten rating on the danger scale from our friends at Skin Deep (www.cosmeticsdatabase.com). It's a known carcinogen in animals and a very likely one in humans, according to the EPA and the Agency for Toxic Substance and Disease Registry (ATSDR)—both government agencies. Yet the stuff is in almost one-third of our products and two-thirds of the bath products made especially for kids, and—you guessed it—it's also in your body wash.

It's the same story for most scrubs as well. For some reason, body scrubs are a favorite candidate for greenwashing, so be extra careful when you choose the brand—it's always apricot-this, sugar-that, eucalyptus-warm-salt-super-slimming blah-blah. Furthermore, scrubbing at your skin is a sure-fire way to make it more easily penetrable by the other chemicals in the product. And it's not just 1,4-dioxane. Parabens, fake fragrance, and all the usual synthetic sinners are in these cleansers and scrubs.

Good thing that this is the absolute most populated clean product section. There are pure sugar scrubs and olive oil soaps and a variety of great options from the Dr. Bronner's pure-castile collection, so there is just no reason to rip at your skin every day; it's yet another part of the cycle that leads to only more products with unreasonable price tags, and unspeakable chemical content.


## Body Lotion

Obvious point No. 1: your skin's your biggest organ. Obvious point No. 2: the skin on your body covers way more ground than the smile lines around your eyes or the dimples on your butt. Whatever you're moisturizing with is being used in much higher quantities and for much longer periods of time. Obviously, then, you should take extra care in choosing one that will love you back in the form of healthy, touchable skin (without any nasty surprises later).

Most basic moisturizers have the same few ingredients. Glycerin, petrolatum, mineral oil, dimethicone, aloe, methylparaben, alcohol, synthetic fragrances, sometimes dyes, and other things we can't pronounce. Many also contain some form of propylene glycol, which is often second only to water on the ingredient lists. That's because it's an effective and inexpensive humectant, which absorbs well and helps draw in moisture.[2] If you've poked around online, you've probably seen it on a lot of natural-cosmetics blacklists. People cite scary factoids about propylene glycol—it is, after all, the same stuff they make antifreeze out of—and point to reports that say it's a strong irritant that should be washed off immediately upon contact.[3] (Confusing advice if you're talking about a moisturizer.)

Of course, these stats aren't revealing the concentrations found in cosmetics. The CIR says all of these ingredients are safe in concentrations of up to 50 percent; the FDA, meanwhile proposed a ban on them in 1992 (the ban did not pass).[4] Problem is, as a consumer, you can't know how much of these chemicals are being used. They're petrochems, so by definition they're not clean from a sourcing perspective. They were also shown to do damage to rats' livers and kidneys in lab studies, and are a known irritant to some people's skin.[5]

So here we invoke "Why bother?" once again—since there *are* plenty of fabulous moisturizers out there that don't double as the stuff they use in fog machines.[6] When you're looking for a good moisturizer, there are a few things you want to check for. First, look for a pure moisturizing agent like shea butter or oils like coconut, olive, or jojoba. Next, there needs to be a humectant—something to attract and lock in moisture. In conventional products, glycerin is used, and it can be here, too; just make sure it's the vegetable variety. And while you're bothering with this annoying post-shower step—seriously, body moisturizing is such a drag, isn't it?—you might as well go anti-aging at the same time and get a lotion that contains green tea catechins or grapeseed extract, too.

## Sunscreen

We know sunscreen is good for you. After all, it protects you from skin cancer, right? But there are some pretty serious concerns around some of the active chemicals used in sunscreen. Oxybenzone is an endocrine disruptor, which can lead to certain types of cancer in women.[7] Not only is it readily absorbed into the body—a 2008 study showed it to be present in the urine samples of 97 percent of the twenty-five hundred test subjects, with higher levels in women and girls—it helps other chemicals in as well.[8] Sunscreen guidelines are also misleading, though new labeling requirements are in the works: SPF ratings refer only to UVB rays, which is cute because, while UVBs do cause sunburns and skin cancer, UVAs also cause skin cancer, not to mention the kind of sun damage that ages us prematurely.[9]

People also feel safe when they throw on their SPF 45, and so they stay out in the sun longer—only increasing their risks, since nobody's really applying the stuff thick enough or often enough for it to do the job properly. And, frankly, even if the active chemicals *were* safe, we wouldn't want you lathering the stuff on because it's filled with a host of other chemicals (like all the ones we already covered in moisturizers). Oh, and guess what? The estimated 4,000 to 6,000 tons of sunscreen that comes off our bodies and into the world's oceans each year is also killing our planet's coral reefs.[10]

But don't panic. This information initially sent the two of us spiraling. In fact, we procrastinated doing sunscreen research because our brains were imploding: how could everything we believed be flipped on its head? Dr. Andrew Weil—whose books and website are go-tos for us—keeps things in perspective when it comes to sunscreen. While he very clearly recommends (as we do) physical blockers over chemical sunscreens, he does say on his site that he sees "the threat of skin cancer as far greater than any theoretical risk posed by the chemicals sunscreen contains." Weil also confirmed that the greatest danger of sunscreen is the "false confidence" it gives people. With this and other input, we have managed to boil things down to a pretty simple formula for you.

1. For starters, we all need some sun on our bodies and you will learn in the next chapter just how important vitamin D is, especially in cancer prevention. And since we're almost all D deficient, we actually encourage *casual* sun exposure, and even some intentional exposure on your arms and legs and wherever else you feel good about showing.
2. If you are the burn-in-two-seconds girl, we think you should mostly avoid the sun as your ancestors did and wear protective clothing (wide-brimmed hats are chic, anyway). When you can't avoid exposure, or for those who have extended outdoor activities planned, there are some good clean sunscreens on the market that use physical blockers (i.e., they sit on top of skin, not allowing the sun to penetrate)—titanium dioxide, and zinc oxide—which provide what is called *broad spectrum* coverage, meaning UVA and UVB protection. You'll need to reapply these often, which can be annoying.

## Deodorant and Antiperspirant

Deodorant was an early controversial cosmetic: way back in 1990 a study was done linking aluminum—the sweat-blocking ingredient in antiperspirant—to Alzheimer's disease.[11] Yikes. Then in 2004, when everyone still crossed themselves up and down, swearing parabens were safe, British researchers discovered trace amounts of the preservative in tissue samples from women with breast cancer.[12] People quickly pointed the finger at deodorant, given the armpit's proximity to the breast. A subsequent study in 2005 put aluminum in the breast cancer

hot seat, too, saying that it can interfere with estrogen receptors—adding that the disproportionately high incidence of cancer in the upper, outer area of the breast provides "supporting
evidence for a role for locally applied cosmetic chemicals in
the development of breast cancer."[13] While the National Cancer
Institute says there is no conclusive evidence linking these and
other ingredients to breast cancer, there's no conclusive evidence to disprove such claims, either. Reassuring?[14]

There are a few other heavy-hitting toxics in most deodorants as well: triclosan is a powerful endocrine disrupter that is
stored in body fat; the ever-confusing talc (correct, the stuff in
baby powder that used to be contaminated with asbestos but
now apparently isn't—yet is still thought to be potentially
harmful); and propylyne glycol (yet again), that sort of sketchy
favorite that might be linked to kidney and/or liver damage.[15]
Not to mention usual suspects like dimethicone and fragrance.
Your average drugstore deodorant likely features several, if not
all, of these.

While nobody wants to be a sweaty mess, the truth is that antiperspirant by its nature is kind of bad: any sweat-blocking
agent, like the very effective aluminum, needs to be small
enough to really get into pores. There's also a serious non-
chemical reality to face: sweating is one of the body's natural
cooling and detoxification methods. So, please, don't think a
Botox shot in your pits is the miracle solution, either. If you're
sweating so profusely that you would consider having that
"natural" poison injected into your sweat glands—an increasingly common procedure—you might want to see a doctor first
about possible causes for your condition. (But be careful when
they give you a slip for industrial-grade antiperspirant; we'd
like you to get to root causes here, not bandaids.) You may

have an overactive thyroid, adrenal issues, a liver problem, anxiety, or a host of other factors that lead to the serious sweats.

We can finish by saying this was hands down the hardest thing to give up and replace. But after trial and much error, we found a deodorant we adore that works well, smells good, and doesn't contain any nasty chemicals. It's in "The Body Guide."


## Perfume

Go figure: the world's first known chemist was a woman. As told on an ancient Mesopotamian cuneiform tablet, Tapputi was her name and perfumery was her discipline. She did it by distilling flowers and oils, and she wasn't alone: in 2005, archeologists discovered what appears to be a full-blown perfume factory, also from the Bronze Age, but this time in Cyprus.[16] See, before it became the chemical concoction we know and love, perfume had many historically relevant incarnations: it was central to religious ceremonies, was used medicinally, played substitute to bathing, and even served as a murder weapon when it was used to poison a French duchesse (death by skin absorption—now, if that isn't proof of what we're talking about . . . ).[17]

The first "modern" perfume, which blended oils and alcohol, was created for the Queen of Hungary in the 1300s, but France ultimately took center stage—Napoleon himself was a major scent enthusiast, using as much as two quarts of the stuff each month, according to lore.[18] It wasn't until 1920 that a French perfumer decided he could make jasmine and rose sing more beautifully together with the introduction of aldehydes, creating the world's first synthetic perfume, and still its most popular: Chanel No. 5.[19]

As we know, the fragrance industry, on top of being self-regulated, is not required to list ingredients on products, thanks to trade-secret laws. This is why all of your products simply say "fragrance." Aside from the phthalates and the weird animal secretions, lab tests on some perfumes have shown tens to hundreds of known neurotoxins, synthetics linked to cancer and birth defects, as well as waste disposal chemicals.[20] You know, like toluene, that solvent that also goes in nail polish and has been linked to liver damage, respiratory issues and spontaneous abortions in women exposed to it at their factory jobs.[21]

Warning: brief, preachy interlude ahead. If you're armed with information, but you still want to get manicures and dye jobs and whatever else, we hear that. The important thing is that you should be allowed to make a choice for yourself based on facts. But when it comes to perfume, that decision affects everyone: the baby you're breastfeeding, your boyfriend, your mom, strangers with serious allergies, and everyone else in the elevator. Finding the right scent is hard enough, so we know that seeking out ones that don't rely on dangerous chemicals is going to be a bit of a bitch. But, honestly, people managed for thousands of years before Chanel No. 5 showed up. Most perfumes are simply mimicking what nature has given us, after all.

## Shaving Creams, Wax, and Depilatories

How many of you have, at some point in your hair-removal careers, had an unfortunate reaction to shaving, waxing or, dare we even say it, *Nairing*? Maybe a rash, weird bumps, or something ingrown that turned cystic. The truth is all forms of hair removal—ripping from the root, shaving, or (ew) "melting"— can aggravate skin, sometimes in very delicate girl spots.

The weird smell of hair-removing creams—thanks to the understudied active potassium thiogycolate—may be enough to deter some of us, but if not, there are always their harsh chemicals. On top of the actives, two things you are sure to find in these depilatories are synthetic fragrance and the ever-controversial mineral oil. We know fragrance comes in everything, but please don't let that desensitize you—it's bad news, and we're talking about areas close to your reproductive organs, your lymph-node-laden armpits, and your long-ass legs. Mineral oil is equally unsavory, aside from being a petroleum-derived eco-beast and a possible pore clogger, it's been known to cause tumors in mice that were injected with it, and is suspected to have caused increased rates of both lung cancer and melanoma in a group of aerospace workers with high rates of exposure to the stuff.[22]

Commercial shaving cream, though, might be even nastier. A quick glance at the ingredients of a brand we all know lists: fragance, quaternium-15 (a formaldehyde releaser), 1,4-dioxane, butane (linked to allergies, irritations, and cancer), BHT (linked to lots of things, including brain damage), and more. And this list is from a "sensitive skin" formula.

For you girls who've stuck to waxing despite the pain, cost, and inconvenience, bless your brave souls. Waxing is generally less offensive than the alternatives—even many store-bought kits contain far fewer chemicals. Still, double-check ingredients, whether you do it at home or in a salon, because *any* toxins will be more readily absorbed due to the heating process and the raw skin.[23] You should also steer clear of the new trend at high-end salons that offer to numb you before the procedure. These numbing creams are extremely dangerous. Like maybe deadly dangerous, and the FDA released a report saying as much in January 2009: they can cause irregular heartbeats, seizures, and comas due to absorption into the bloodstream, and two women in their twenties died after topical application.[24] Finally, and this is important too, to soothe your skin, most estheticians will want to slather you in creams. Don't let them. Bring your own pure aloe or some other clean alternative with soothing properties, and use that instead.

## Stretch Mark Creams

Oh, stretch marks. Many of us have had you since our very first teenage growth spurt, while others acquired you during those savage weight fluctuations of our twenties. And for you who thought you were home free? An estimated 75 to 90 percent of women are left with striae (their fancy name) post-childbirth. We're not *that* awesome at math, but by our calculations, this means pretty much all of us will get stretch marks at some point. So how about a little self-acceptance, yeah? Besides, your lovers probably don't give a crap about them. The good ones are just happy to see you naked.

Stretch marks are not as simple as people think, though, and when it comes to getting rid of them, it's like the common cold: there is no silver bullet. Depending where they appear, how long and deep they run, and the tone of your skin, stretch marks run the gamut. If your skin is darker, the silvery brown lines could be more apparent than the white ones on alabaster complexions, but women of all skin tones have given up bikinis after having kids (shame!), or shied away from daytime sex (criminal!) while looking for solutions.

The reason they are so impossible to get rid of is the tears happen in the dermis, which is below the epidermis, the layer we think of as our actual skin. They are, in fact, scar tissue, and as severe burns illustrate, the deeper the damage, the harder it is for scars to heal. Also, contrary to popular belief, stretch marks are not just a consequence of weight gain; they also happen from weight loss, and muscle gain (dudes get them a lot on their pecs, for example); and they are affected by hormonal changes, as well as certain medications, like the topical steroids widely prescribed for other skin conditions.[25]

The often-expensive creams on the market that claim to get rid of striae will do no such thing, and we know because we've tried them. Predictably, they also feature all of the same infamous ingredients as your average moisturizer. We spent a small fortune on one well-known brand—with its overhyped Pal-KT-TKS—and it sure as hell didn't get rid of our stretch marks. There is also some evidence that Retin-A can help reduce the appearance of stretch marks (see Chapter 5 for our full take on Retin-A).[26] Some lasers promise to take care of them, and Alexandra dared to find out . . .

---

### LASER QUEST
#### Alexandra Tries To Zap Her Stretch Marks

"It's a question of light," I explain to the nurse as an assistant pops into the room with a camera. This is a little embarrassing. They want to take a "before" picture of the stretch marks on my chest, and so far, they're having a little trouble seeing them. My stretch marks are the textural kind. They never announced themselves in red or purple flare, and they only appeared a few years ago—long after my growth spurts were over and not with a pregnancy. I motion toward the window and the women follow me and alas—as soon as natural light hits me—there they are.

The nurse lets out a perceptible "oh" and asks gently—if there ever were a gentle way to ask such a thing—whether I used to be over-weight. Um. No? I've stuck to your basic five-pound fluctuation for ages. She seems perplexed and expresses concern for my marks if I get pregnant—I'm about ready to put my shirt back on.

I realize I am being a bit dramatic. I know that even the world's best bodies are stretch-marked, and when I see them on others I think, "No big deal—cute even." But we're never as kind to ourselves. So when the opportunity arose to diminish mine with the fanciest new laser treatment in town, I jumped. And since my town is Los Angeles, I'm in good hands.

The very candid Dr. Alexander Rivkin is quick to say there are no guarantees with this particular treatment. While his honesty inspires trust, I don't want to believe him! He tells me that the medical world still does not have the full picture on the causes of striae, which would explain why there's no clear prevention strategy. He surmises it's part genetics, part hormones, and definitely too-quick-too-much skin stretching. While many questions remain, Rivkin is able to explain to me why stretch marks have been so impossible to beat, even with lasers. "Microscopically speaking, a stretch mark is the disruption of a large band of skin. And because the damage has gone so deep, there can be no healthy skin there to help rebuild it." I finally get it: because lasers work by causing targeted damage that triggers skin to rejuve-nate itself, if there's not enough of that healthy surrounding skin, both below and beside, it just won't happen. The lasers also need to go deep enough, which until recently, they couldn't do.

And so here I am, about to meet the Deep FX—the first laser that may just go deep enough. This, in combination with the more super-ficial but very popular Active FX, add up to what's called the *Total FX* experience.

The machine looks and sounds like a vacuum cleaner from the '70s, and I've opted out of numbing cream. To my great relief, however, the pain is totally bearable, and the nurse maneuvers the awkward piece of machinery with relative grace. I've already tried every form of hair removal out there—laser *with* numbing cream, waxing, electrolysis—and on the pain scale, this rates far lower.

The first few post-treatment hours are tinged with a stinging pain and a visual to match: it's a sunburn. In pixels. A bad one. The pain passes quickly, though, and the next few days are a weird little game of watching myself heal. It's not a pretty sight, but I'm transfixed, con-stantly checking to see if I notice improvement—which at this point is impossible since it's a red, bumpy mess.

The careful inspection goes on for at least a month. Maybe longer. In the first week there is peeling and the fresh, pink skin below looks definitely improved, I think. It's still pretty hard to tell. But as time passes, and the redness fades—not completely mind you—it seems that my marks are still there. Yup, still there. And to boot, two months later, I still have mildly sunburned cleavage.

At three months, there remains the slightest discoloration, mostly noticeable after a hot shower, which might mean that the skin is still healing and potentially repairing itself (and my stretch marks). But, honestly, at this point, I've stopped caring. I really can't tell if there is any change at all in the marks. And given that I'd probably have to do this again a couple of more times to get any real results—as the kind doctor had told me—that could mean a year in and out of boob burn, not to mention costing a small fortune that I don't have.

And so, my quest ends. Will the technology get there one day? Probably. Will I try again? Not likely. (Though if you're still game, do as

I did and find the best place in your town. This is not a procedure to skimp on.) My post-laser M.O. is that in life there are things we can change and things we have no control over. It's more rewarding to put our energy into the former, and try your best to either accept (or at least ignore) the latter. And to get a few really nice bras.

---

## Cellulite Treatments

Freaking cellulite. The conventional wisdom for preventing cellulite sounds a lot like the conventional wisdom for everything else: not smoking (slows circulation), drinking lots of water (flushes out toxins—though it's up for debate whether toxins, in fact, cause cellulite), and having great genes. All good advice, sure, but if you're reading this, you're probably not fourteen, don't have a time machine, and are already living with some dimples you wish weren't there.

Research about the causes of cellulite is inconclusive and debated. We'll spare you a trip to the peer-reviewed-journal boxing ring and say this: cellulite is the result of how your body stores fat, and that's something you can't control. As a general rule, women store the stuff in their boobs, hips, thighs, butt, and—evil of all evils—their upper arms. Whether that fat looks dimpled or smooth seems to be determined by the pattern of connective tissue beneath the skin that holds your fat cells together.

Most guys have nice crosshatched holders that keep the cells in place. The cruel joke is that women's fat tends to be held with column-like structures, making it easier for fat to poke through. Skinny bitches as well as the more zaftig among us— same deal. Same columns. Same cellulite.

Dr. Mehmet Oz said on *Oprah* that "you can't put a cream on and get inside the fat cell."[27] Makes sense. So topicals and fancy treatments can't fix your problem. What they can do is increase tissue swelling that temporarily improves the look of the dimples (others, meanwhile, help it contract, for a tighter look). And don't think you can lipo your way out of this one. Studies show that liposuction can severely worsen the look of cellulite. So why are we telling you all this? It helps to know what you're trying to get rid of before you charge another hundred bucks to the card and say a prayer to the cellulite gods.

As far as the nasties in cellulite creams are concerned, these ones really run the gamut, from the hyper-scary kind that rate eight to ten on Skin Deep's database, to ones that earned a gentler three. Look yours up before you buy, and if it's not there, look up the ingredients. What you'll notice is that cellulite creams use a dizzying number of different ingredients (probably because none of them work), and most of them are not good for you.

A popular active is caffeine. Caffeine is thought to reduce swelling around the fat, constricting blood vessels and making your skin appear smoother. Some bogus studies even say caffeine can help melt fat, reducing a half-inch off your butt in six weeks. One widely cited study that shows caffeine benefits cellulite was paid for by cosmetics companies that sell these products.[28] Another says it might work when used with ultrasound therapy to help carry the caffeine deep enough into the skin to work, but even then the effect would be temporary.[29] Either way, we're not convinced. The reason so many companies use caffeine is probably because it's a relative of aminophylline, another ingredient that used to be thought of as a cellulite-busting silver bullet[30]—that is, until it came out that the studies saying that ingredient was so awesome were done by someone who was marketing a cream containing this magical ingredient.[31] Aminophylline is also prohibited in cosmetics in Canada and elsewhere. The FDA says it can cause allergic reactions and that it's concerned about the use of this ingredient in cosmetics.[32] Too bad the FDA hasn't done anything about that, though. Creams with caffeine in them should not be used while you're pregnant, no matter how natural the other ingredients are. Caffeine and fetuses are not friends.

So what to do? There are pricey treatments like endermologie and VelaSmooth, which can work for a little while, but Dr. Rivkin also provides a healthy dose of skepticism when it comes to these: "People do seem to like them, but it's hard to know how much of that is placebo. They definitely don't work for everyone." Ultimately, we think the best approach is getting over it and tweaking with things that can improve the look of the skin. Clean self-tanners or body bronzers are a good bet, as are clean tightening lotions that can make it less noticeable. Also, while exercise can't make it go away, increasing your muscle-to-fat ratio—which isn't to say weight loss, which can just make it *more* visible—can help skin appear more taut, if not airbrushed-perfect.

### Self-Tanners

Let's be honest, dirty chemicals aside, there are probably a few good reasons to avoid self-tanners: like, say, Tara Reid. Or stained clothing, dark armpits, orange hairlines, and streaks. That said, we did find one—yes, a whole single one—clean product, and it was from Lavera. And we found an almost-clean option that we loved for our legs. (Confidential to natural cosmetics companies: fill this hole in the market.)

The primary active ingredient that puts that tan in the bottle is called dihydroxyacetone (DHA), and despite the creepy name, it seems to be fairly harmless when applied topically. DHA is just a simple carbohydrate—the "bad carb" if you're on a diet—that can be derived from natural sources, like beet and cane sugar. Discovered by accident in a German lab nearly a century ago, DHA reacts with amino acids in the top layer of skin, creating a pigment called melanoidins—these resemble melanin, the real tan that happens at a deeper level (in the dermis).[33] It's been approved for use in cosmetics since 1973 and has a fairly clean public track record.

Here's the catch we do know of: a 2007 study done by Germans found that exposure to sun shortly after applying the self-tanner makes you way more susceptible to free-radical damage—like, 180 percent more.[34] Therefore, if you still want to use the stuff, you have to be extremely careful to avoid the sun for at least a day after application, because with that kind of potential damage, you might as well just tan.

The other catch is that self-tanners tend to wear off pretty quickly (they slough off with your skin cells) and require frequent reapplication on large surface areas. So you might not need to worry about DHA, but in conventional self-tanners, you want to be wary of the preservatives, fragrance, dyes, penetration enhancers, and chemical byproducts.

Take one look at the stuff: the color, the shine, the intense burned perfume smell, the way it coats your skin in color *before* the DHA has had a chance to act on it. DHA is colorless and takes a few minutes to work, but because cosmetics companies want to give you that immediate satisfaction—seeing a difference right away upon application—they load it with crap that gets all over your towel and clothes to make you think it's working right away.

A word about spray and mist tanning: even the FDA warns against this method. It's not that there is necessarily a big difference in ingredients between the creams and the mists (though, honestly, do you think the staffers on *Sunset Tan* know what the eff is in there?); they also use DHA as their active. It's just that the FDA is not sure it should be inhaled.

## Real Tanning

Nobody's saying to grab the Crisco and pull out your mom's old reflector from the garage, but if you haven't noticed, more and more stories are coming out about the benefits of vitamin D. Meanwhile, a whopping 77 percent of Americans are seriously vitamin D deficient.[35] It's been claimed all over the media that the complete villainization of the sun over the last twenty years is in part responsible for this universal deficiency (it's also created a *huge* anti-sun cosmetics market). An SPF of just 15 blocks 99 percent of vitamin D absorption (and the American Academy of Dermatology recommends a *minimum* SPF of 30).[36] This is not to say that our fears about the sun are wrong: it will age your skin prematurely and can cause skin cancer. Point blank. But being less of a sun-Nazi, and getting a little bit of unprotected exposure on your arms and legs, between five and fifteen minutes a day, depending on your skin type, may be good for you. Just don't overdo it; don't do it at all if you burn easily or have any history of skin cancer in your family; and, if you care about wrinkles, don't tan your face.

## THE BODY GUIDE

### Body Washes and Soap

*Pangea Organics Bar Soap*
These are just the perfect bars of soap, made from a variety of yummy, all-natural ingredients. With nine different ones to choose from, creative combos include: Tunisian Olive Oil and Coconut, Green Tea with Mint and Rose Petals, and Canadian Pine with White Sage.

*Dr. Bronner's Magic Soaps*
These are the OG in natural soaps. Bronner, a German immigrant whose parents were killed in the Holocaust, came to America and started making soaps at home more than sixty years ago. He was quite the character and wrote messages on the bottles promoting his unique life philosophies. He died in 1997, and the bottles are still covered in his eccentric ravings. These vegetable-based liquids and bars come in a variety of simple formulations, like almond, peppermint, lavender, and more. In celebration of the company's sixtieth anniversary, it released a USDA Certified Organic line.

*Ren Moroccan Rose Otto Body Wash*
We love Ren because it brings so much class to the clean market. From the packaging to the product, it's pure luxury. However, there's a price tag on that feeling, as we well know. This

---

### DELICIOUS DIY BODY SCRUBS

We're not the most regular exfoliators, which means we've both dropped a pretty penny on some fancy pot of scrub only to see it sit in the shower past its prime. If that's you, we have two ideas: (1) get yourself a good set of scrubby gloves or even just a washcloth, or (2) experiment with making your own scrub. Here's what you need:

- an exfoliating ingredient such as brown sugar or sea salt (choose your coarseness, or combine them)
- a skin-friendly oil, such as jojoba, coconut, or olive oil
- essential oils if you're into smells (we like vanilla—who doesn't?)

Mix these ingredients however it pleases you (this really isn't chemical engineering), for a fraction of the cost, in the quantity that suits your needs. Done.

---

body wash, which uses one of the most expensive essential oils out there, smells and feels incredible. Even the mainstream is onto it: *InStyle* magazine rated it the top body wash of 2009. There's also a **Moroccan Rose Otto Sugar Body Polish**; if you really have some money to burn, it's a total treat.

*Jurlique Body Exfoliating Gel*
This is yet another delicious product in a lovely bottle (yes, we are influenced by packaging). The exfoliating ingredient here is a walnut shell powder, so this is a gentler scrub and is good for more sensitive skin. Other key ingredients high on the list are green tea extract and turmeric, which is known for its anti-inflammatory powers.

Your Body

183

## Body Lotions

*Dr. Hauschka Rose Body Lotion*
Ignore the unappealing mustard hue (it beats fake dyes), and slather it on. You'll find it unusually light and easily absorbed— a rarity with naturals. The rose fragrance is delicate and feminine, not the sometimes geriatric version, but if you're still not a fan of this flower, you can try out the quince or lemon versions.

*Elemental Herbology Skin Drink*
They call this their "summer" lotion because it's light and loaded with watermelon, cucumber, and grapefruit—decidedly refreshing extracts. But we like it year round for its delicate smell, quick absorption, and antioxidants. It's gentle enough for Siobhan's super-reactive skin and garners questions like "Why are your legs so soft?" Works for us.

*Juice Beauty's Green Apple SPF20*
*Antioxidant Body Moisturizer*
As the name indicated, this body cream is all about everything in one. It's packed with antioxidants like vitamin C, resveratrol, and green tea, and thanks to its non-nano titanium dioxide it also offers good sun protection. We find the initial smell a bit too tangy, but it fades fast. We're fans of the Green Apple Extra Firming Body Moisturizer as well.

## Sunscreens

*Aubrey Organics Natural Green Tea Protective Sunscreen*
You know you can trust Aubrey, and this sunscreen clocks in at

the best price point (less than ten dollars). It has healthy oils, green tea antioxidant power, and 10 percent titanium dioxide to block that sun out. You have to reapply, but the payoff is you're blocking UVAs *and* UVBs.

### Soleo Organics

This company probably puts out the most legit natural sunscreen on the market. It won't even use titanium dioxide (which you may recall is slightly controversial from an inhalation angle, though it does not penetrate skin), so this is all good old zinc oxide. The EWG's made this sunscreen its top pick out of the one thousand reviewed. It doesn't get cleaner than this.

### Lavera Sun Block SPF 20

The latest formulation of this sunscreen is compliant with the new European regulations on UVA rays (go team Europe!). Lavera is serious about its broad-spectrum protection—the website even talks about UVC rays, which last time we checked didn't even penetrate our atmosphere.


## Deodorant/Antiperspirant

### Lavanila The Healthy Deodorant

This is the Cadillac of nontoxic deodorants. It's expensive, it looks good in the shop, it smells good, and lo and behold, it works. We promise. While it has its own lovely smells (we like the grapefruit-vanilla best), Lavanila seems to have mastered a formula that kills your own stench—as opposed to just masking it. Hooray to that.

## DIY DEODORANT

We came up with a little formula that did a decent job on our pits. We mixed some baking soda—known for its odor-killing powers, as any refrigerator can testify—with our favorite essential oils and carried the concoction in an empty mineral makeup case. We applied it just like we do mineral makeup, using one of those short, wide kabuki brushes. It does require fairly frequent applications, but we found that the baking soda really helps neutralize odor.

### Weleda Sage or Citrus Deodorant

We love Weleda, and its spray deodorant was one of the better ones we came across (seriously, though, it's *that* hard to find a good one). However, we noticed that after several weeks of wear, it stopped fully covering us on our stinkier days. If odor isn't a big problem for you, this product might be the perfect choice, though.

### Tom's of Maine Deodorant

We'd like to be able to fully endorse Tom's of Maine. In our hippie homes, we knew about Tom's way back in elementary school. We really like the company's long-lasting roll-on deodorant, but there's one drawback: one of the ingredients is propylene glycol. We've already said that it's not clean, though not the worst, so we'll leave the choice to you. We still think Tom's is way better than any mainstream brand, and while we didn't cover teeth in this book, you should know that Tom's is the king of natural dental care. The end.

## Hair Removal: Shaving Creams, Waxes, and Depilatories

### Tom's of Maine Shaving Lotion

We're happy to report that this Tom's product is entirely clean and its toothpaste-like tube makes it easy to store. The cream itself doesn't propel out of a bottle foamed for you, so you'll have to lather up a quarter-inch between your hands, then slather it in. It makes for a really close, even shave, with no skin reactions or redness.

### Dr. Bronner's Organic Shaving Gel

Stop the presses, the raddest soap brand of all time now has a shaving cream as part of its new USDA Certified Organics line. It comes in the same great classic scents as the soaps and works like a charm.

### Moom Organic Hair Remover

Neither of us are wax girls, mostly because we're not into that kind of pain and hate waiting for hair to grow back in. Still, this super-clean sugar wax from Canadian company Moom comes highly recommended and can be bought online. If you're going to go the home route, sugar waxes like this are less of a mess because you can just wash the stuff off (your body, your floor . . . wherever you may get it). The formula here is sugar, lemon, tea tree oil, and water. That's it.

### DIY Waxing

You might be thinking, hey, I can make that myself. Well, of course you can. Combine one-half cup of water with one-half cup of lemon juice and a cup of sugar, heating the mixture it to keep it at around 230 to 240 degrees. When it begins to darken, take it off the stove and let it cool to about to about 110 degrees before painting it on in strokes. Once it hardens, rip it off. Obviously don't try this if you're a waxing novice, and even if you're not, supervision is highly recommended.

## Perfume

Perfume is far too individual for us to tell you what to use. So instead we're opting to list some brands that carry a variety of wonderful fragrances. You're going to have to explore these on your own to find the right match for you. **Tsi-La** is a favorite in the natural market, and offers a wide selection of perfume that smells like sophisticated scent blends, as opposed to just glorified essential oils—which we happen to also love; **Intelligent Nutrients** carries lovely aromatics that carry different properties (we like the sensual one and the one for focus—as perfume, though, not as medicine); **Jurlique** does a series of yummy, blended essential oils; and **InFiore** offers the ultimate in hippie-chic with its line of solid perfumes in stunning gold cases. We also love **EOV (Essence of Vali),** the signature smell by the amazing Valerie Benis, and Café Noir or Pamplemousse by **Dawn Spencer Huriwitz.**

### DIY Perfumes

Since we like to keep home formulations uber simple, we were quite pleased with this one for fragrances. Use a high quality, organic vanilla extract (yes, the kind you use in cookies)—this works well as a base because it's sweet, delicious, and already contains alcohol, a key ingredient in perfume. Then, blend in your favorite essential oil. Alexandra uses a cedar one in about equal parts to the vanilla (which makes for a warm, woodsy smell)—carrying it around in one of those lovely little, dark glass John Masters bottles she had left over. (Dark bottles are a good idea because they protect the concoction from light, and it will keep longer.) There is a world to choose from here, so get creative and make something that is uniquely you. If you don't like vanilla (you're weird, who doesn't like vanilla?) you could try a different extract, like almond, or even straight vodka as your carrier.

## The Impossibles: Stretch Marks and Cellulite

There's really no silver bullet for these afflictions, so we're not going to lie to you and tell you to go buy something that doesn't work. The best advice we can give is to moisturize and massage and exercise. Also, both afflictions (if we want to call them that) are less noticeable on evened-out and tanned skin, so that's an easy bet. Feel free to use anything off our moisturizer list (**Juice's firming cream** is a good one for cellulite) and we found one self-tanner we love (**Tarte's CelluFight**), that we think you might love, too. But if you're not afraid of going for something a little heavier, we suggest using healthy oils, like almond, sesame, coconut, jojoba, or argan. Pure shea butter is great, too. **Dr. Hauschka** makes a **Blackthorn Body Oil** geared for stretch marks that we love, and **Weleda's Skin Food** cream is perfect for trouble spots because it is so rich and nourishing. In the lifestyle chapter (Chapter 10), we will also introduce you to Ayurvedic self-massage, a relaxing practice that is amazing for skin maintenance.

## YOUR BODY AT THE DRUGSTORE

Target strikes again, carrying the **Weleda** deodorant and both the **Lavera** self-tanner and sunscreen. Otherwise most drugstores are going to be limited to your more basic body washes and lotions, though in those categories there's a decent selection. **Burt's Bees** again, here, has some nice products as does **Yes To**. Most places also carry the liquid soap from **Dr. Bronner's**, which we use for our bodies, our hands (and occasionally our dishes). The Alba line features lots of nice and clean body products, including sunscreen, and its mother company **Avalon Organics** has plenty of goods as well. **J. R. Watkins**, a solid, clean line, is available at Walgreens and drugstore.com.

## Self-Tanners

### Lavera Self Tanner

This product is clean enough to be used on your face, too, if you so desire. It contains some good oils as well as some great antioxidants. Well done, Lavera. Just remember not to go in the sun for twenty-four hours after application.

### Tarte CelluFIGHT Self-Tanner

This two-in-one wears and feels and works like a pricey conventional self-tanner. It builds slowly with repeated applications, and goes on colorlessly—which helps reduce streaking. We also did feel a little more taut in our tushies.

*Josie Maran Bronzing Argan Oil*
Not exactly a self-tanner, this bronzing oil is great on the body, too. Rub it on arms and legs or even chest and cleavage, for a nice glow. Maybe don't wear white that night, though.

# 8

## Your Nails

There's something counterintuitive about nails. We tend to forget that, like hair, they are extensions of our body. Unlike hair, though, they're affixed to our skin and can absorb whatever gunk we put on them. Don't believe us? Lest we remind you what your bare toes look like after months of consecutive pedis with Russian Roulette–red polish—dried out, brittle, and, yes, stained. If your nails weren't porous, there wouldn't be a stain, now, would there?

Our nails, like our faces, directly reflect how we treat them. In fact, in certain traditions like Chinese medicine, nails are used as an indicator of overall health and can be a useful diagnostic tool for illnesses that may be lurking in the body. Even the father of medicine Hippocrates said so, and that was twenty-four-hundred years ago.[1] This makes sense because our nails grow out of us, specifically out of the skin folds at their base—or "roots"—so when we eat nothing but Cheetos, don't get our vitamins, or, you know, irritate our nail beds with harsh chemicals, guess what happens? Our nails look bad.

## MEET YOUR NAILS

Nails grow in a process called keratinization. Root word: keratin, that protein that's in our hair and the top layer of our skin. As we produce more keratin, it pushes out and flattens the dead protein, forming nails. Those half moons under the skin are called lunula, and they're part of the nail matrix. The matrix is sensitive and remembers all the bad that happens to it, so those little white spots you get sometimes are not calcium deposits or signs of zinc deficiencies or whatever your mother told you they were. They're more like bruises: memories of a trauma in the nail matrix—like being pressed on too hard during a manicure, or, you know, coming into contact with the nasty stuff in nail polish.[2]

The pinkish part, meanwhile, is white; the rosy hue reflects tiny blood vessels underneath the nail. The white part—that pretty bit we fake with French manicures—is where the nail separates from the skin at our fingers and toes tips.[3]

So they're made of dead cells. But the matrix they grow out of, the cuticle, and the nail bed are all very much alive and require all the things the rest of our bodies need to survive. If you've ever been in a swimming pool, you know how soft nails become when they're wet. That's because they can absorb up to 25 percent of their weight in water from a single soak.[4] Now think of the basic mani. We soak multiple times, softening the nails and making them more porous, then we pile on the strengtheners and varnishes and acrylics and glues that contain some of the most toxic ingredients on the beauty market. We're lucky we still *have* nails after all that abuse.

FDA literature states explicitly that "under the law, cosmetic products and ingredients, including nail products, are not subject to FDA premarket approval authority, with the exception of most color additives."[5] Yes, we're repeating ourselves, but these things, like the toxic chemicals in your beauty products, take a second to sink in.

## Nail polish

The big-three chemicals commonly found in nail polish are toluene, DBP (a phthalate), and our good friend formaldehyde. Toluene makes the polish brush on smoothly, DBP is a plasticizer, and formaldehyde is a hardener. DBP, one of the phthalates banned in Europe, has shown in studies to be an endocrine disruptor that causes underdeveloped genitals in male fetuses.[6] Toluene is also widely banned and restricted in other countries; and formaldehyde is classified as a known carcinogen in humans.[7] Check Chapter 3 for a refresher on these three. Cosmetics companies and their buddies in regulation will tell you that the amounts used are so small and cannot pose health risks, but since amounts are not required to be listed, there's really no way to know what that means. Meanwhile, the effects of long-term and repeated exposure are also not known. So despite multiple bans worldwide, these chemicals are still used in many conventional polishes in the United States. They probably also have something to do with the fact that nail polish is classified as hazardous waste in California.[8] As in, you're not supposed to put your polish and remover in the regular trash.[9]

Meanwhile, official FDA policy states that "by law, nail products sold in the United States must be free of poisonous or deleterious substances that might injure users when used . . .

[and] labels of all cosmetics . . . must include a warning statement whenever necessary or appropriate to prevent a health hazard that may occur with use of the product."[10] We call bullshit on this, obviously. Otherwise, your pedi would come with warnings like cigarettes. So take it from us, since we can't take it from them: the stuff in your nail polish is not stuff you want in your bloodstream or your lungs.

The irony is that these chemicals are part of a thriving market that doesn't even need them. There are exceptional alternatives out there, which is why it was such a huge deal when OPI announced it would change its formula to exclude toluene and DBP from its polishes (there wasn't formaldehyde in there to begin with—it was in their strengthener, though).[11] That salon favorite faced mounting pressure from the badasses at the Campaign for Safe Cosmetics, and around 2007 switched it up.

Still, we encourage you to read the superfine print on all your beauty products. Not to be a total wet blanket, but even some polishes without the big-threes are not completely clean; there's a chance we know even less about their replacement ingredients. So the same rules apply here, as with other beauty products: got a hot date? Paint away. Getting a weekly mani? We've got some ideas coming for you.

## Strengtheners

Then there's nail strengtheners. These typically contain formaldehyde, which hardens the nail but also can cause nail lifting and allergic reactions in some people. Take any bestseller in the category marketed as "protein" or "vitamins" for your nails. By now these kinds of claims are probably as absurd to you as they are to us, but we'll hammer home the point: your nails are dead protein that cannot be strengthened by you painting chemicals on them. They may benefit from having chems painted on them in the sense that it cosmetically reinforces the nail—like varnishing a table can seal in a paint job or protect the grain of the wood. Except you're not made of wood. Aside from formaldehyde, most strengtheners also contain a host of other unpronounceables. Then often at the end of some lists there's "protein," "keratin," and, um, "calcium."

## Mani-Pedis

If you, like us, have no intention of giving up your mani-pedi, there are some options. You can learn to do it yourself with nontoxic polish (boring), or you can find a salon that is less toxic and dirty than most (fun). First, you don't want to go anywhere with whirly footbaths. A bazillion reports and newspaper articles will tell you this: they are havens for bacteria that can cause stubborn and peep-toe-unfriendly infections. Also, look for places that truly sterilize the equipment they use. If it's not clear, ask. If the answer is unconvincing, leave. And if you're pregnant, run.

As a guiding principle, if it reeks of "nail polish smell"—a highly volatile mix of sometimes-toxic chemical fumes, which are as bad to inhale as they are to pour into your skin—it means the salon is not being properly ventilated. "The solvents used [in nail-salon products] are formulated to dry very quickly, which means certain chemicals also evaporate almost immediately. Once they evaporate, they end up in the air you breathe," says Rebecca Sutton, a senior scientist at the Environmental

Working Group. "We should certainly be concerned about exposure to these chemicals. We are constantly exposed to other chemicals as well, and we don't necessarily know how they are interacting with each other and what the long-term effects of exposure can be on the human body."[12]

Also of growing concern to the EWG (and to the rest of us) are the health effects these chemicals may have on technicians whose livelihoods require daily exposure to such fumes. We spoke with researchers at the Northern California Cancer Center (NCCC), who are working on the first large-scale study of cancer risk in the nail salon workforce. They are also doing some exploratory measurements of occupational exposure to certain chemicals in nail salon workers in California. While the study is ongoing, we are eager to see what they find and trust that this will spark a greater national inquiry into the effects of long-term exposure to volatile organic compounds (VOCs).

Recently, we've both discovered the chicness of a buff manicure. It's clean and put-together looking, and hey, if it's good enough for P. Diddy . . . Plus, you don't have to worry about chipping (and cancer), and the benefits are manifold. The rubbing increases circulation and while we couldn't find a scientist to corroborate our observations, we noticed that our nails seemed to grow way faster. Also, since it smoothes ridges, it can stop nails from splitting. Ask your manicurist to skip the chemy lotions she applies before buffing. That's just a lazy shortcut. For a real buff, a buffing board on its own is all you need for high shine. It makes for a nice pedi, too, but if you've ever walked around New York in flip-flops in the summer, you understand the impulse to regularly polish your toes.

If you want to polish, and your salon only carries Essie or some other big-three brand, bring your own, and don't forget your basecoat. We recently went for pedis and were fussy about the polish choice—there's a list of nontoxic ones we like at the end of this chapter—but then the technician reached for another brand of basecoat. It was a little awkward to ask her to take it off, but we did. A toxic basecoat defeats the whole purpose.

Tough call on all the other crap they slather onto you, too. You can assume they are full of things you no longer use, and we're not about to propose you show up with your own caddy from Whole Foods. One option is to find an eco salon in your city. If yours doesn't have one, or if it's a pain to get to, then make sure the polish is clean and consider forgoing the other stuff altogether—get the foot massage without lotion, and insist on a pumice callus remover instead of the chemical ones. Certain chains, like Dashing Diva, now have essential oils on offer in addition to creams. Remember, you don't have to be insane about this, but every little bit you put on counts and adds up, so choose carefully.

## Fake Nails

You know where this is going. Suffice to say that fake nails applied in salons using mysterious powders and glues are probably not going to be great for you, but we understand the appeal. Done well, they look pretty. When Siobhan used to be a nail biter, she'd get them to help her grow hers out. Of course, once they soaked them off with acetone, her nails were so ravaged and dry that they'd break off when she so much as patted away at her BlackBerry for a few seconds, defeating the purpose altogether.

But what are they? Fake nails are generally made out of acrylic polymers. When rats inhaled this stuff in lab tests, it caused nose and eye irritation, lung hemorrhage, and degenerative changes in the liver and kidneys.[13] Cute, right? We'll spare you the chemistry lesson, but after the reaction is completed to form your lovely new fake nails, traces of monomers sometimes remain and can result in irritation, allergic reaction, and painful swelling of the nail bed.[14] What's worse, the crap they use to prime the nails so your acrylics stay put often contains something called methacrylic acid (MAA), which, in response to cases of poisoning, now requires child-safety packaging. The industry-backed scientists at the CIR determined in 2002 that MAA is safe in cosmetics when used as directed, as long as skin contact is avoided.[15] Maybe someone should remind the CIR that your nails are attached to your skin. And that the people applying the gunk also have skin. And that, yep, there's even skin under your nails.

If that doesn't deter you, though, maybe fungal infections will. These are common with fake nails because things get trapped, and they proliferate. Nail fungus is harder to get rid of than red wine stains on white jeans.

Bottom line: don't wear fake nails.


### Nail Polish Remover

Most nail polishes' active ingredient is acetone, a highly flammable chemical that helps things dissolve. It's commonly used to remove fakies or polish, and in high enough quantities it can cause a scary list of health effects, from skin irritations and lightheadedness to stomach problems and shorter menstrual cycles.[16] It can be absorbed into the blood through your skin, and even more easily through your lungs.[17] Women regularly exposed to it in high enough quantities—that nice lady who does your nails, say—have reported getting their periods early.[18] But even if your period is normal, you can count "drying out your nails" as a fairly reliable side effect. And before you pat yourself on the back for knowing better than to use acetone removers, may we remind you this: if you don't use acetone, you're using some other nasty crap. In fact, just recently, the FDA announced the voluntary recall of a non-acetone remover, "enriched with gelatin," when two people complained that they'd been burned by it.[19]

## Cuticle Softeners and Removers

"Cut or push back?" The million-dollar question has a simple answer. Your cuticles are there to protect the area right beneath it (which the nail grows out of), so if you use a chemical cuticle remover, or cut them all off, you're increasing the risk of infection, and possibly damaging the nail matrix. This is entirely avoidable, of course, by leaving your cuticles alone. To keep them supple and pretty, get a nail oil and apply it with a Q-tip after you shower in the morning. It's amazing what a difference that alone can make.

## Callus and Corn Removers

Calluses are something we sort of think you should learn to love. If you have them, it probably means you work out, go to the beach a lot, or walk around barefoot. But we get the whole not wanting to rub your rough feet against the lucky person in your bed thing, so some thoughts. Calluses are, like corns, your skin trying to protect you from pressure and injury. They form on areas that get lots of friction (like your baby toe against your pumps) and serve a purpose. Over-the-counter treatment lotions are not advisable for obvious reasons: they're loaded with high-concentration acids, petrochemicals, and sometimes rubber, and they can burn the heck out of your skin.[20] If your calluses hurt for some reason, and you can't whittle them down with a pumice stone, you should see a doctor, who might remove some of the dead skin with a knife. Do *not* cut them off yourself.

## THE NAILS GUIDE

*Polish*

*Priti Nail Polish*
Polish by this nontoxic nail care pioneer is the fashionista's best bet. The packaging is cute, the color selection covers all the basics, as well as trendy and saucy seasonal options, and it wears like a charm. When you're done with it, her polish remover works nicely, too.

*Zoya Nail Polish*
This was voted the longest-wearing nail polish by *Women's Health* magazine—not bad for a polish that's cleaner than

most. We really liked it for the concentrated color and range of choices. One caveat: this puppy goes on thick and can look a tad plasticky with two coats. We opted for one, and our pedi lasted so long you could see the nails growing out.

## Remover

*Honeybee Gardens Odorless Nail Polish Remover*
This stuff is acetone and fragrance free. It truly smells like nothing, and it does a decent job. It wipes off polish with a few cotton balls, and while it leave nails a little dry-looking (there's alcohol in it), it was nothing a little oil couldn't fix.

*Suncoat Naturals Nail Polish Remover*
This is the cleanest and most effective option we tried. It also washes off when you're done, and since it's biodegradable, it won't poison our friends in the sea. Dab it on with a cottonball or toilet paper, leave it alone for couple of minutes, then rub it off.

## Nail and Cuticle Oil

*Dr. Hauschka Neem Nail Oil & Nail Pen*
This stuff comes in a bottle or a nifty, handbag-friendly applicator and absorbs quickly into the cuticles and nail. After our last chemy manicures left our nails splitting, we found this conditioned the nail and softened ragged cuticles. Neem is also a natural antifungal and antimicrobial.

NAILS

## Hand and Foot Lotions

*Jurlique Purely Age-Defying Hand Treatment*
This sort of redefines the idea of a high-performance hand cream. It's a potent, nongreasy moisturizer, so it's great to keep in your desk at work (no slippery typing fingers), and contains licorice, which has something in it called glabridin that Japanese studies isolated as a natural lightener.[21] You know what that means: more even skin and faded sunspots.

*Weleda Skin Food (used as a foot cream)*
This cult favorite is amazing: cheap and highly effective on any dry areas (elbows, cuticles, hands—we've even used it under our eyes). It's exceptional for calloused gym feet as well. Slather it on, put on some cotton socks, and call it a night. It helps cracked heels, rough calluses, and skin peeling.

## DIY

NAILS

*The Buff Mani-Pedi*
May we propose a challenge? Go without a polished mani for a month and see what happens. In the meantime, go buff: skip a chemy shine cream and just get a good board, and once a week (not more) gently buff your nails in one direction only. Do not go overboard or you'll thin the nails. If it starts to burn, you've gone way too far.

*Vegetable Oil Nail Soak*
We told you earlier that your nails can absorb up to 25 percent of their weight in water. That also means they can lose that wa-

---

## YOUR NAILS AT THE DRUGSTORE

Several drugstore brands seem to have made some effort to clean up their nail lines. Hopefully others will follow **OPI**'s lead here and go "three-free" (that's formaldehyde, toluene, and DBP free). For now, **Revlon**, **L'Oréal Paris**, and **Sally Hansen** are also all cleaner options than the ones containing the three nasties.

---

ter: plumped up after you do the dishes, dried out after. To remedy this, do a weekly soak with an organic veggie oil, which can be even better than nail creams because it doesn't contain alcohol or other drying agents.[22] Wash after, but don't scrub. You just want to lose the excess.

*Biotin Supplements for Nails*
Cauliflower and lentils both contain the nutrient biotin. It's part of the B complex, and supplementing with it could be great for nails. A Swiss study showed that after six months, many people taking biotin supplements had remarkably thicker nails, and experts concur![23]

*Milk Soak for Hands and Feet*
Milk has lots going for it. Its lactic acid can gently remove rough skin, and it's considered a good moisturizer, too. Pour a cup of milk into a cup of water (add in some olive oil if you're really dry), and heat it slowly, being careful not to burn it. Let it cool slightly, and then soak your hands or feet in it for about five minutes.

NAILS

### Pumice Stone Callus Remover

The best way to remove calluses is the old-fashioned way. Soak your feet in a bucket of water and apple cider vinegar for at least ten minutes. With the skin nice and soft, grab a basic pumice stone and chisel away. Remember, though, that calluses are natural protectors from friction—they stop you from slipping around in your stilettos and on your yoga mat—so don't go crazy.

### Cuticle Softener

Lots of different pure oils work well here. We like neem, but the smell takes some getting used to. Jojoba and olive oils work well, too. Just rub it into the nail bed and cuticle vigorously after a shower, leave it on a few minutes, then wipe off whatever excess there is. Do this once a week.

### Lemon Age-Spot Removers

The acid in lemons is strong enough to get rid of some age spots, but it'll take some dedication. Daily for six weeks, rub fresh squeezed lemon juice or slice onto the spots, and watch as they miraculously disappear. Do this at night, though. Lemon increases sensitivity to sun.

NAILS

# 9

# Your Diet

Some starlet once said she wouldn't put anything on her face unless she'd be willing to drink it. We agree—and we've already introduced you to some products to fit that bill. But we'd be doing you a great disservice if we just left it at that. Most of this book has been devoted to explaining (over and over) why putting the healthiest of things on your skin, that sponge of an organ, is the key to beauty. But of course, that story is not complete until we look at what you're intentionally ingesting as well.

If we've heard it once, we've heard it a thousand times: we are what we eat. While that notion has been around for centuries, recent science has really driven home the crucial role diets play in our overall health. Health, you may have heard, has a little bit to do with how good you look. In fact, many of the biological indicators for beauty (nice skin, shiny hair, rosy cheeks) are outside manifestations of good health. And in an over-simplified, animal kingdom kind of way, those signifiers increase our mating appeal.

## MEET YOUR DIET

In other words, if you want to look and feel your best, you can't just switch to a paraben-free cleanser, eat hotdogs every night, and expect to glow. Ditto the idea that eating no fat and lots of edamame is a prescription for beauty: it might make you skinny, but it won't make you shine.

What will? The most luminous, healthy women we know have incredible diets. That is not to say they live a life of deprival, nor do they feast only at gourmet, organic restaurants, spending a fortune every time their stomachs growl. It's about balance and eating whole foods—not processed crap loaded with preservatives that are nastier than the ones in your shampoo. It's also about joy, which, as you'll see in the next chapter, is as important as this food business. A healthy, balanced diet full of delicious (and nutritious) foods is your secret weapon. We promise, nothing could be kinder to your looks.

When it comes to eating, the rules are similar to the rules about skin care: the more unadulterated the product, the better. If you like the taste of apples, you should eat an apple, not a toaster pop with jellied "apples" in the middle. Same goes for chicken. If you like chicken, eat chicken. But don't eat hormone-packed, water-pumped coldcuts. If you hate anything green, you're shit out of luck, though. You have to eat your greens. But top yours with something you do enjoy, like a bit of cheese, or a homemade dressing, or, our favorite, lots of olive oil, salt, pepper, and garlic.

Eating well is generally good advice, but particularly for skin. "Nutrition is the cornerstone to building and repair for every cell in our bodies," says celebrity nutritionist Paula Simpson. Read that sentence again, would you? *Every* cell. And while healthy skin cell turnover occurs every three to five weeks—powered by your amazingly nutritious diet, of course—this process slows down as we get older. "If we are not supporting our bodies with the critical nutrients to promote healthy skin cell turnover and protection, then we know this will stimulate accelerated aging of the skin." Ouch.

Our skin, as we've mentioned, is not just our largest organ, but also one entrusted with the unpleasant task of elimination. It's not supposed to do a ton of heavy lifting; that's what our bowels are for. When you don't eat well, your digestion gets messed up, and when your digestion gets messed up, your skin acts like a temperamental teenager. Additionally, says Simpson, "Toxins, if not eliminated or neutralized, can accumulate in our bodies, particularly in fat tissue. Chronic toxicity coupled with poor nutritional status will definitely reflect in your skin, hair, nails, and eyes."

Fear not, however: we are not going to tell you that French fries and chocolate in moderation are going to make you ugly. We will, however, tell you that an unbalanced diet loaded with sugar, preservatives, dyes, and bad fats is beauty enemy number one. Eating crap—or just *not eating enough*—starves your cells of the nutrients they need to be healthy, burdens your body, and prevents you from going to the bathroom enough. (We promise we'll stop talking about bowels now.)

We realize this might not be exactly the way scientists would phrase it. They love telling you that food has nothing to do with your acne or your sallow complexion. Like, sure, it might be hard to prove in a study that people with balanced diets tend to have an insanely hot glow to them, and that people who actually eat vegetables look (and feel) better in their sixties than their meat-and-potato sisters, but empirical evidence, when it

## A FEW WORDS ABOUT SUPPLEMENTS

When it comes to getting the vitamins and minerals that we need to look—ahem, *feel*—our best, we agree that food is the best source. We've read the same studies you have that supplements are a bunch of hooey. With that said, there is a strong body of research that claims certain vitamins are extra-good for illness prevention, and that some cannot be adequately consumed from food sources alone. In those cases, we advocate pill popping. But do your homework, get as high-quality supplements as you can afford, and most of all, pay attention to your diet.

comes to vanity pursuits like nice skin and fewer wrinkles, is king here.

We have both spent years experimenting with our diets to figure out what suits us best and have enjoyed consulting experts of all stripes along the way, including ones a little outside the mainstream. Take Ayurveda, that ancient Indian tradition that says you are what you eat. It's the foundation of Deepak Chopra's best-seller *Perfect Health*. According to Ayurvedic tradition, there are three main types of energies (*doshas*) in people. Most of us are a combination of the three, with different dietary needs based on our type. When the fiery *dosha*, called *pitta*, gets out of balance, as one example, it can show up in the form of eczema, acne, and prickly rashes. Eat cucumbers for a week (along with other cooling, calming foods) and presto! No more rashes. That's a gross oversimplification, but the point is that sometimes food really is our best medicine.

Are we getting too flaky for you? We thought so. All we're

trying to say is that there are plenty of traditions other than the one most of us grew up in that says food has a pretty direct impact on how we look and feel. It doesn't mean you'll stop reading studies every year that say acne isn't caused by pizza, or premature skin aging isn't caused by the toll processed foods take on our bodies. Everyone loves a good story that disconnects us further from the foods we eat. But if there's one takeaway from this chapter, let it be that we shorten that gap.

## Inflammation and Your Skin

If there's a buzzword in health research right now it's "inflammation." It's been fingered in rheumatoid arthritis, Alzheimer's, heart disease, cancer, and chronic diseases of all kinds, including those of the skin.[1] It's also the immune response to infection and injury: you hurt yourself and your immune system uses inflammation to fight off the bad guys. This is the good kind of inflammation. That neat trick aside, some diseases trigger inflammation when there is nothing there for the immune system to fight off. That is the bad kind. Chronic internal inflammation is the kind that can be life threatening, and one of its triggers is—you guessed it—food. When we eat too much saturated (animal) and trans fat, our bodies overproduce free radicals. These "steal" electrons from healthy cells, which can lead to inflammation.[2] Meanwhile, other inflammatory foods, such as sugars, prompt a cascade of hormones that essentially tell your body it is stressed the eff out, which can aggravate acne. If you eat the right things, however, that chain of events is reversed. Good food equals reduced inflammation. Bad food equals increased inflammation.

Is inflammation the root of all evil when it comes to our skin? "We know that inflammation is the precursor to many chronic conditions that include the skin," says Simpson. "Inflammation can accelerate skin aging by destroying the structural integrity of skin, reduce dermal blood flow, and increase the incidence of chronic skin conditions." We'll take that as a yes.

What else causes inflammation? Oh, everything. Allergies, stress, toxins, over consumption of booze, caffeine, smoking, sugar . . . um, being alive. There are studies that say overexerting yourself at the gym can accelerate inflammation, and other studies that say exercise can reduce it.[3] While some of the triggers are hard to avoid in modern life, inflammation can be calmed by adhering to an anti-inflammatory diet, which docs like Andrew Weil and others advocate.[4] The fact that it's loaded with delicious food choices makes it a pretty easy sell for us: blueberries, omega-3-packed fish, garlic, ginger, sweet potatoes, walnuts, turmeric, whole grains ("brown" bread doesn't count), egg whites, spinach, red wine in moderation, to name only a few. Also good are monounsaturated fats like olive oil, avocado oil, canola oil, and peanut oil. Yum! High-quality fish oil supplements are also a great bet for anyone with inflammatory skin issues (acne, rosacea, aging), as is zinc, which has helped some acne sufferers because it speeds up wound healing and wards off infections, while calming inflammation. Make sure you take it on a full stomach, though.

### Sugar, Empty Carbs, Starchy Things, and Your Skin

When we talk about sugar, we aren't just talking about the white stuff you put in your coffee at breakfast. We also mean anything that zips through the body quickly, spiking insulin: white flour, corn, pasta, maple syrup, baked goods, fruit juices, sodas, sweetened iced teas, anything containing high fructose corn syrup and on and on and on. While they're not nice to your body, the thing about sugar is that it really likes to make itself known on your skin, too.

There are a few ways sugar shows up in your skin. The first is the most obvious: it triggers inflammation, which, as we discussed above, increases the signs of aging, including wrinkles. It can also worsen acne.

"Glycation" is kind of a buzzword in beauty right now. You'll see it used in skin care ads: new potions that promise to reverse the glycation of skin (and thus make you look forever twenty-one). In skin, it is the process by which simple sugar molecules latch onto collagen without an enzyme there as a buffer. This creates a series of reactions that contribute to the formation of wrinkles and, according to the writings of Dr. Nicholas Perricone's *The Perricone Prescription*, can increase the leathery appearance of some skin.

Researchers have also started looking at the role insulin can play in acne.[5] When we eat things that spike our blood sugar (think white bread, pasta, peanut M&Ms), our pancreas starts pumping out insulin.[6] This hormone behaves similarly to male sex hormones and increases oil production by stimulating the sebaceous glands.[7] And when those glands overproduce at the same time that skin cells slough off too quickly and inflammation increases, guess what happens? To beat this out, focus on an anti-inflammatory diet loaded with antioxidants, clean proteins like salmon (or ground flaxseed and walnuts if you don't do fish) and you should be well on your way to clearer skin.

## Protein and Your Skin

The first thing anyone will ask you when you tell them you're a vegetarian is, "But what do you do for protein?" Which is funny because the truth is it's very difficult to not get enough protein. Very few of us are actually deficient.[8] Protein is crucial for a number of reasons, the simplest of which is that protein is needed to repair cells, make new tissue, and maintain healthy tissue. So when you don't get your protein, the motor that powers your body's ability to fix itself is a little low on juice.[9]

We're going to pretend that no one eats (drinks?) powdered protein anymore and focus on real food. There are two main ways to get these amino acid chains we call protein: vegetable sources and animal sources. Under the former are beans, grains, a few nuts. The latter includes animal and fish flesh of all kinds, as well as eggs. Here, your best choices come from the former, which offer a less concentrated amount of protein and lots of other nutrients, meaning you get more bang for your buck—a little vitamin C or fiber or unsaturated fat to go with your protein. In the animal category, you'd do best to stick to fish (but make sure you're not choosing overfished ones, or ones high in mercury) and eggs (the whites themselves contain a ton of protein, though the yolks are loaded with good vitamins and minerals—your call, but may we suggest cage free?). Both pack a protein punch, taste good, and have other health benefits to recommend them. As for other kinds of meat: red meat is mostly bad for you, and the livestock industry alone accounted for 18 percent of global carbon emissions in 2006— compared to the auto industry's 13 percent.[10] This is pretty straightforward stuff, right?

## Alcohol and Your Skin

Speaking of which . . . perhaps you have noticed that every couple of years there is a new study saying a drink a day is great for you, and then another saying it ages you and gives you breast cancer. Well it appears as though unlike cosmetics, where we don't want anything to do with their poisonous ingredients—the "poison" in booze really is in the dose. Everyone we consulted agreed that a glass of alcohol a day is not just okay, but awesome. Not only could it reduce the risk of heart disease, it also chills you the hell out at the end of the day.[11] (Stress-busters are beautifiers, as you'll see in the next chapter.) So never mind the fact that we have trouble believing there are not better ways of preventing heart disease. If the pros think we should enjoy a cocktail a day, then a cocktail it is. The trick is limiting it to one.

Ironically, most of the benefits of booze—countering inflammation, preventing heart disease, calming you down, relaxing your blood vessels—sort of flips on its head with the second drink. That's when its face-reddening, dehydrating, puffiness-inducing, glycation-promoting properties kick in. Excess alcohol can also hurt your liver (duh), and we all know our liver is responsible for clearing out the toxins that make us look like garbage. Overtax your liver, and what happens? Bad skin. Too much alcohol can also interfere with your body's ability to absorb calcium—which can lead to osteoporosis—and can dull your complexion. We have no idea why this last bit is true, but look around: it totally is.

Finally, booze contains sugar, and if you skimmed the section on sugar above, take a moment and go back a few pages.

This applies to alcohol, too. So if you're drinking cosmos or tonic water or anything blue or green or fuchsia—please tell us you're not—then you're looking at even more bad stuff. We're not telling you not to drink at all—every girl needs to let loose once in a while—but for the love of all things great, stick to wine, basic spirits, and simple mixers. And when you're contemplating your third drink before dinner, think back: can you remember the last time you had three drinks before dinner? Yes? Then it's too soon to do it again.

## Teas

Using tea therapeutically can be pretty amazing. Got a tummy ache? Reach for peppermint. Anxious? Chamomile. No tea has a better and more beautifying rap than green tea, though. Its benefits are very well documented for disease prevention and for providing a kinder, gentler form of aging, mainly because it's loaded with antioxidants called polyphenols. Make sure you get a good quality tea, though, and organic is better—that way you can be sure you aren't canceling out the benefits of green tea with the toxic pesticides used to grow it.

There is also interesting new research about white tea. White tea, it turns out, is also packed to the gills with antioxidants, which are as good for your skin as they are for the rest of you. A recent study showed that white tea prevented the breakdown of elastin and collagen, which, of course, is a good thing.[12] It did so by stopping the offending enzymes from doing the damage in the first place. (These are the same enzymes that are associated with inflammatory diseases, so your health gets a boost, too.) We're daily green tea devotees, and we encourage you to experiment. You can't go wrong drinking the stuff.

## AGUA! THE FINAL WORD ON WATER

You should drink plenty of purified water or water-heavy, sugar-free beverages such as green tea every day. Given all the controversies surrounding bottled water—like, if it's just tap water, what's the carbon footprint of Fiji, and where do all those bottles go?—we've taken to activated charcoal filters like moths to light.[13] You should, too.

## Antioxidants and Your Skin

We tend to think of antioxidants as the skin gods' second chance, but they work best as a form of prevention and maintenance. Of course, since our skin is in a constant state of flux (and—sniff—degeneration), it's never too late to start loading up on them. If you haven't already, it's time to meet your new best friends.

First off: all antioxidants are also anti-inflammatories.[14] Memorize that fun fact. It's important. Second, antioxidants work by neutralizing free radicals and oxidative stress before they can cause harm to our cells. Harm like cancer, and harm like shitty skin. Free radicals come from pollution, stress, alcohol, bad diet, toxins of all kinds (including the ones in your old shampoo), smoking, and public-enemy-number-one, the sun. The cruel joke is that free-radical generation can also be stimulated by overly exertive exercise and by a host of other things, including simply getting older.

To counter the effects of our vices, nutritionists strongly advise *daily* consumption of antioxidants. If you're the kind of chick who really eats her eight to ten servings of nutrient-dense fruits and veggies every single day of your life, then you are our hero, and you don't need to take an antioxidant supplement. But realistically, on a daily basis, that is harder than finding perfect jeans.

"This is where supplementation can help bridge the gap between poor nutrition and optimal health," says Simpson, who has her own line of anti-aging nutritional supplements called GliSoDin Skin. She thinks—and we agree—that food is king, and supplements should not be thought of as a quick fix. It seems many people think it can, though, which probably accounts for the fact that antioxidants are a $2 billion a year industry for vitamins C, E, and beta carotene alone.

## Vitamins and Carotenoids

When we refer to vitamins, we mean the kind you get from your food, for the most part, not the kind you take in pill form. Among stellar antioxidants are vitamins C and E, and carotenoids like beta carotene (the stuff in carrots) and lycopene (the stuff in tomatoes). We already looked at how topical C might boost collagen formation and enhance skin's protection from the sun, but getting enough in the food we eat is also critical to fighting free radicals and maintaining a healthy immune system. It can help ward off all kinds of infections—not just colds. You can also supplement with C, but go for the powdered form. It's most readily absorbed and a daily dose might even help rosacea sufferers with their pinkish glow. Carotenoids, meanwhile, are other great antioxidants. Dr. Oz, in *YOU: Being Beautiful*, even went so far as to say that tomatoes—which are loaded with vitamins C and A, and lycopene—

might be as good as acai and goji, those trendy, expensive antioxidants you couldn't stop hearing about for a few years.

Unless you're looking for a boost in antioxidants, you're better off getting your C and your carotenoids from fruits and veggies. It's not that hard to do, folks. Couple of carrot sticks, some tomatoes, and a handful of most fruit or leafy greens several times a week and you're set. (Also those rumors about too much beta carotene turning you orange are true—it's not toxic to overdose on carrots, but it's not recommended or necessary, either.) C has a proven track record, especially when it comes to beauty, but it is oversold as a cure-all. As for E, it's a little harder to get it exclusively from food sources. It's a good antioxidant, though, so experts suggest you take 400 IUs a day in supplement form, but make sure it's natural E, not synthetic.

Then there's vitamin $D_3$—the hottest vitamin since $B_{12}$. There are interesting (and misinformed) headlines all the time about this wonder vitamin's health benefits, but the fact that more than half of Americans are vitamin $D_3$ deficient is cause for concern, because it's a vital nutrient capable of doing all kinds of cool things in our bodies. Let's try to set the record straight.

$D_3$ is produced in the skin when it reacts with UVB rays. That is why people will tell you that to get the $D_3$ you need, you should spend time getting unfiltered sun exposure for ten to twenty minutes a day, depending on your skin type. (More exposure time is needed for darker skin, which contains a natural SPF.) The problem with that is that the sun is just not strong enough in most parts, and so taking it in pill form is increasingly recommended.[15] It sounds like it might be worth our while, because $D_3$ does two very impressive things. One, it slows cell growth, which helps prevent and fight cancer, because that's what cancer cells like to do (reproduce way too quickly, that is). It also scans your DNA for errors, and kills them.[16] Experts say that almost every cell in the body has vitamin D receptors, which means it has the ability to affect an endless number of its functions.[17] Research is ongoing. Like E, vitamin $D_3$ is hard to get enough of from food. Experts recommend supplementing with 1,000 IUs a day. Make sure you get $D_3$, the kind our skin makes naturally, not $D_2$.

## Omega-3 Fatty Acids

Back to omegas. Yeah, we know you've heard of them, but do you know why they're so stellar? Omega-3s are an essential fatty acid with hundreds of strong studies backing up their health benefits, from boosting brain function and easing arthritis, to preventing diabetes, heart disease, and breast cancer. There is even one study that says omega-3s help reduce asthmatic symptoms. Really, what don't they do?[18]

There are also countless studies attesting to its other important function: making you look amazing. Kat James, the beauty expert and author of *The Truth About Beauty*, writes that the "effect on my own skin from fish oil was nothing short of amazing. Within a couple of months of starting this regimen, my skin literally 'forgot' that it had been continually irritated. . . ." We have also found that omegas have reduced breakouts, balanced dry skin, and given our hair a lustrous shine. We even know someone who had chronic conjunctivitis, whose bloodshot eyes were kept at bay as long as he took his fish oil.

You can get a decent amount through your diet. Wild Atlantic salmon, mackerel, sardines, some algae, and ground flax seeds are good choices. (You don't need to eat a fillet daily; three fist-sized portions a week should do the trick. For ground flax seeds, a tablespoon a day sprinkled on salads or your cereal works.) Bear in mind that overfishing is a growing concern, and the environmental implications of eating fish are inescapable. If you want to chow down with a clear conscience, you're going to want to stick to stinky sardines. And if you're vegetarian, go for algae, soybeans, or flax. You can also get an extra boost in supplement form. We both take ours daily and stick to high-quality, low-food-chain sources, like those by Nordic Naturals. It helps beat out bad moods and stress, reduces inflammation, strengthens nails and hair, and generally makes you more gorgeous with every dose. Stock up.

## Coenzyme $Q_{10}$

Another good antioxidant with some solid backup from team science is $CoQ_{10}$. It appears in topical form in some cosmetics and is widely available on the shelves of natural food stores in supplement form. $CoQ_{10}$ scavenges for free-radicals that lead to wrinkles and might mitigate photo aging, and in one study, its use appeared to have a 51 percent decrease in biological aging in mice.[19] The jury's out on how well it works, but if you're bulking up on antioxidants, this is, for our money, a better bet than some of these trendy ones that come into vogue and cost a fortune and are hard to find. Take anywhere from 60 to 200 mgs a day.

## Resveratrol

Unless you live in a cave, you have probably heard of resveratrol, an antioxidant found in the skin of red grapes. It came to most people's attention after a Harvard University study pointed to the supplement's ability to extend lifespan and protect aging mammals' brains without any negative side effects.[20] Other people heard about resveratrol because of well-publicized studies, claiming everything from mice to worms to yeast live longer when taking it.[21]

Simpson explains that "resveratrol is a polyphenol antioxidant famously found in red wine and is believed to be the factor behind the 'French paradox.'" That is, being able to eat and drink whatever you want and still look lovely and lithe (and heart-disease-free). "It is also a component of pomegranates, blueberries, olive leaf, and other 'wonder foods,'" she goes on, "believed to reduce oxidative stress from free radicals and so prevent the symptoms of aging."

Let's get this straight: we get to drink red wine, eat a baguette with butter, and look like a hot French chick well into our sixties? Well, not so fast. While resveratrol is, indeed, an antioxidant, the problem, says Simpson, is that the amount of it in fruit isn't enough to have much of an impact. (And to get any positive effects from the resveratrol in wine you'd have to drink twenty-four bottles a day.[22]) So while there are countless benefits of eating plenty of fruit and drinking moderate amounts of wine, getting enough resveratrol isn't one of them. What about supplements? Is this pill the magical elixir of youth? Mayyyyybe. There are certainly compelling studies out there, but we're not running out to buy the latest promise in a bottle just yet.

Simpson's advice, meanwhile, is to eat a healthy diet, and supplement it with a commercially available antioxidant product. Maybe for you that's resveratrol. For now, we're sticking to the less exotic ones with longer track records, but we're keeping our ears out for more good news. Who doesn't want another excuse to have a glass of red with dinner?

## SHOPPING LIST

If you're going to eat only ten things, eat these.

1. *Tomatoes.* Organic tomatoes are loaded with lycopene, a powerful antioxidant shown to help fight illness and cancers of all stripes. Works well with green tea and broccoli, too.
2. *Green tea.* Put simply, people who drink green tea have about a dozen health advantages over people who do not, from cancer prevention, to longevity, to nicer skin (okay so the last bit might not be in a study, but we buy it).
3. *Broccoli.* Well-documented for its aid in the prevention of several cancers, cell detoxification, repairing sun-damaged skin, bone health, eye health, and immunity.
4. *Salmon.* Can we be lazy and just tell you to take our word for it? Short version: anti-inflammatory omegas, B vitamins, heart-disease prevention, cholesterol-lowering power, great skin. *Et cetera.*
5. *Extra virgin olive oil.* It's gotta be EV: eat it for heart-disease prevention, its cholesterol-lowering good fats, its antioxidants, and because it's completely and utterly delicious and frankly tastes better than butter. Yeah, we said it.
6. *Dark leafy greens.* Yes, they can be bitter and a little less than exciting at first, but they are loaded with vitamins and iron and can be snuck into meals easily (omelets, pasta, salads, etc.).
7. *Walnuts.* Packed with good fats (monounsaturated), these are awesome for heart health, lowering cholesterol, boosting brain function, and reducing inflammation. A dab'll do ya, though.
8. *Blueberries.* High in vitamin C (which means great for skin), fiber, boosts brain function, anti-cancer powers, and awesome on cereal.
9. *Avocados.* Loaded with cholesterol-lowering power, potassium, folate, carotenoids, vitamin E, and happiness-inducing monounsaturated fats.
10. *Dark chocolate.* Because it's delicious, and it's almost as good as sex. Also, antioxidants.

## TWO INDUSTRIES IN A POD

In many ways, the business of food and the business of beauty are strangely analogous.

While what we eat is certainly *more* regulated by government agencies than the makeup we wear, huge holes in the system and unchecked corporate power have left consumers (and the environment) in shambles. (This is well-treaded territory by writers such as Eric Schlosser, Michael Pollan, and Rory Freedman and Kim Barnouin.) As such, many of us have taken our health into our own hands—diligently reading ingredients labels, choosing farmers markets over supermarkets, reading studies on the effects of our diets, and so on.

Obviously, this is the type of proactive behavior we're advocating—whether we're talking about your dinner or your conditioner. While it's frustrating that there isn't more oversight in place to protect the consumer in both of these industries, there is also something very satisfying about taking charge of our own bodies, especially as women. You don't have to be a bra burner to recognize that we've had a long-ass history of being told that we know nothing about our own bodies. Now onto the last ingredient in this recipe for health and beauty. . . .

# 10

## Your Lifestyle

We know, and have bought into, the product promise for as long as we can remember. Ever since grade school, in fact. It's not our fault: the way these things are sold to us, we'd be almost crazy *not* to think that a bottle or a tube has more control over our looks than we do. Part of not falling for the marketing (or the brainwashing) means realizing that there are things we can do simply, cheaply, and healthily that have nothing to do with furthering a multibillion-dollar business. What if, instead of the eye cream that doesn't work, you begin thinking that five hours of sleep are insufficient? And what if, instead of piling on the luminizer, you break up with your products and hook up with someone you like, instead?

### MEET YOUR LIFE

Unless you've been under a rock for the last decade or two, you've probably heard that stress is bad for you. It's been linked to everything from infertility to heart disease and the mainstream is finally embracing what was once considered the flaky centerpiece of alternative medicine: the old mind-body connection, about which the country's biggest celeb MDs—Mehmet Oz, Andrew Weil, and Christiane Northrup—have been shouting from the rooftops for ages.[1] We'd like to take that mind-body duo and turn it into a threesome, though: call it the mind-body-beauty connection.

Long before we cared about the crap in our cosmetics, we were taking baby steps to reduce our stress and improve our health in other ways. We ditched the gym for monthly passes to the yoga studio, became adamant about our seven (or eight or nine) hours of sleep a night, tried to stop taking work home with us—that kind of thing. Aside from feeling better, we quickly realized that we were starting to look better, too.

In this mind-body-beauty connection, stress is the biggest wellness buster. It's also something of an epidemic: back in 2007 almost half of Americans between nineteen and forty-nine reported feeling frequent stress.[2] And that was before the recession. What's worse, stress is also a very direct factor on the way we look. Because we know you are best convinced by cold hard facts, let's look at a few examples before we get into the more general ways we can reduce our stress and improve our health.

## Stress and Your Skin

### Stress and Skin Repair

*Don't make that face or it'll get stuck like that.* It appears that moms everywhere might have been onto something. Those of us over the age of twenty-five have probably noticed that our most frequent expressions are slowly being carved into our

## IN DEFENSE OF NERVES

But wait! Before we lead you down some path to total anxiety-free living, we'd like to say this: anxiety has its perks. The same thing that wakes some of us up in the middle of the night with streams of going-nowhere thoughts, is also the motivating factor that gets us to work in the morning. Naturally anxious people are believed to be harder workers, better prepared, and generally more thoughtful. Anxiety has historically produced its share of great art, too (like, all of it). So the point is not to pathologize stress or suggest we all spend our days meditating on mountaintops. It's just that most of our lifestyles aggravate what may already be a genetic predisposition— some 20 percent of us are thought to be *born* worriers, exhibiting the signs as early as four months old. And for too many people anxiety is a constant groan, while for others it manifests in extreme swings (like full-blown panic attacks)—these are the cycles we'd like to help you avoid.[3]

faces in the form of fine (or not-so-fine) lines. Of course, it cuts all ways. Too much scowling and your forehead becomes a map of anxiety. Too many smiles, as if such a thing were possible and it's crow's feet for life. Still, there's something decidedly less attractive about the wrinkles that come from frequent frowning, wouldn't you say?

Another way that stress may be blowing your good looks is by hindering your skin's ability to repair itself. Dr. Ladan Mostaghimi, a dermatologist and professor at the University of Wisconsin, has been studying the relationship between skin, stress, and sleep. She mentions a study of people under chronic stress—one subject group was made up of caregivers for people with Alzheimer's—who displayed a delayed capacity for wound healing. "There have also been studies that show delayed wound healing in students during exam periods," she says. But Mostaghimi is quick to point out that it's not a simple causal relationship: "It's important to understand that the effect of stress depends on the type and intensity and duration of the stress, and that's the reason why, even though we have known for thousands of years that stress can make you sick, we still have so many conflicting studies about it." She does, however, know that stress plays an aggravating role in a number of skin disorders, including acne, psoriasis, atopic dermatitis, urticaria (a kind of rash), hair disorders, and cancer.

*Stress and Your Hormones*

We're not going to delve too deeply into hormones; the way in which they impact us is often individual (and complicated). But we will say this: there's a clear link between stress, hormones, and skin. There are also some basic principles that we do understand when it comes to this relationship. Both the stress hormone cortisol and the sex or androgen hormones can play a role in acne and other skin conditions, and their levels can be influenced by stress. Cortisol, which is released during stressful situations, can suppress the immune system, giving certain bacteria the opportunity to flourish, sometimes resulting in some kind of skin flareup.[4] Cortisol and androgens are often cited as acne culprits because they're known to increase sebum production, and some women show raised androgen levels under stress as well, as part of that famous "flight or fight" response. Until recently, research about this stuff has focused on males, and studies seem to indicate that most women do not respond with that same "fight or flight" hormone flood. But as occasional stress cases prone to breakouts, we call bullshit on that.[5]

So how do you know if stress is wreaking havoc on your skin? Well, before you run off for blood work, just think about it. Does your skin look markedly better when you're on vacation? Is your PMS worse when you're stressed? Do you instabreakout when your boss gets on your case? Sometimes, these indicators are pretty clear, though not always. If you suspect a more serious or persistent imbalance in your hormones (as indicated by moods, skin, period, what have you), please get it checked out. Polycystic Ovarian Syndrome, thyroid disease, and adrenal disorders can all wreak havoc on your skin. Same goes for chronic stress and its cousin depression. It's no way to live, and we strongly encourage that you seek out some kind of counsel.

## THE LIFESTYLE LIST

Enough about what stress does. Let's look at how we can reduce it. Consider this lifestyle list as a simple prescription for looking your absolute best. Because unlike pretty little noses and perfect perky boobs, these are things you can control. So don't skimp.

### Get Greedy About Your Sleep

We all know that sleep makes us look and feel better—but do we know why? Well for starters, not enough sleep affects our overall mood, and cranky girls aren't pretty girls. It's a vicious cycle, too. Those of us with anxiety have a hard time sleeping; the less sleep we get, the more on edge we feel, the more grumpy-frowny faces we make, and so on. This is probably one of the worst cycles to be in, and if you're currently stuck there, we have some suggestions coming. Getting yourself into a decent sleep schedule should be at the top of your priority list— right up there with cleaning out your dirty cosmetics.

Sleep also just gives us a nice break from our facial gymnastics; that might sound oversimplified but it's true. The longer you sleep, the more time your face spends not frowning, laughing, and squinting. Pretty straightforward stuff. Chronic lack of sleep will age you in other ways, too. Rats that are entirely deprived of sleep will die within ten to twenty days—that's a quicker demise than starvation. (And you *know* those rats looked like shit, too.) Humans who suffer from an extremely rare sleep-depriving disease known as fatal familial insomnia will die within months.[6] While scientists don't completely understand why they die—there is still so much we don't know about sleep—it certainly bolsters the claims that good sleep is one of the key components of good health.

What we do know for sure is that non-REM sleep, which is about 80 percent of the snooze, is vital to cell repair. Basically, the downtime lets you fix some of what happens during the up time; that rest period enables enzymes damaged by free radicals to be replaced by new ones.[7] It's not a big leap from there to understanding the relationship between getting your Zs and having healthy, younger-looking skin.

Despite all the compelling data, most of us aren't getting enough sleep. The perfect amount varies by person, but the general recommendation hovers somewhere between seven and nine hours per night. Most people report getting only about six.[8] What's more, three quarters of the population say they have problems sleeping.[9] Meanwhile, the quick-fix sleep meds leave you with a hangover so bad it's almost worse than not sleeping at all.

So, if you're serious about sleep, and you should be, you need to make a concerted effort to improve it, while not getting stressed out about it (yes, life is a series of challenges and contradictions). For us, this has meant getting onto an earlier schedule. Yep, turn off the TV and be in bed with a book by 10 p.m. Whether or not it's true that the hours before midnight offer better quality sleep, it sure *feels* true. There is a belief in Ayurvedic medicine that between the hours of 10 p.m. and 2 a.m., when we're not sleeping, we enter an "active" cycle. That means your mind is more likely to start buzzing around again, making it harder to fall asleep. We know it's not for everyone—some people are natural-born night owls—but going to bed early is easier than you think. If you force yourself to get up at 6 a.m. a few mornings in a row (it helps to let light into the room), you'll be ready to go down at 10 p.m. in no time. Or, when you're not partying your face off, just start inching it back a little earlier, night by night.

Also, it's proven that raising your body temperature aids in inducing sleep, whether that's a warm bath, shower, or cup of tea.[10] (Ironically, the best room temperature is on the cooler side—so many rules.) Darkness also helps suppress melatonin,[11] so dim the lights and step away from the TV and computer a good hour before you want to go down. If you're a city girl, get some blackout blinds. The IKEA ones work great, and they're relatively inexpensive. We also think essential oils can help. Siobhan dabs a little lavender under her nose before bed.

Another option is Essence of Vali's sleep potion, which smells so good we would wear it as perfume if it weren't for its slightly narcotic effect. Finally, inhale. Everyone always tells you to "exhale" when you're stressed. You should obviously do both, but the truth is that when we're a little wound up, it's our *inhalations* that get shorter. Focus on making your inhales at least the same length as your exhales, and presto! The mind shuts up.

One last thought: if you're having a really hard time falling asleep, do something else. Turn on the light. Pick up that boring book you promised yourself you'd read. Alphabetize your BluRays. Because nothing begets insomnia like insomnia.

### Exercise, Exercise, Exercise

Like sleep, exercise has more benefits than we can count. We're going to skip the whole weight-loss thing, because that's not what this book's about. Yes, exercise can improve your looks, make your body firmer, beat out anxiety and depression, make you feel accomplished and proud, increase circulation, boost your energy during the day, and tucker you out for bedtime. These are all good things, but there's a chemical component here, too.

One of those chemicals is nitric oxide, which relaxes the walls of your arteries—part of the formula for maintaining low blood pressure. Then there's our friend serotonin: the happy hormone. Exercising releases serotonin, which is why we feel energized and psyched about life after workouts. Also, as long as you're not exercising right before bed, it's proven to help sleep, too.

So you're less stressed, and your ass looks better—but what's exercise really doing for you in the beauty department? Well, it's getting the toxins out and that's a key to great skin. This happens in a few ways: it improves circulation, stimulating lymphatic movement (the system that rids the body of toxins); it oxygenates cells; and, finally, it makes us sweat out the bad stuff. Perhaps most importantly, though, it gives us that natural glow that chemical cosmetics have yet to duplicate in a bottle. Oh, but how they try.

### Invest in Love and Marriage (But Mostly Sex)

Speaking of glow, the kind that comes from sex is no myth, either. First there's good old sexual flushing that happens to up to 75 percent of women and can last for a few post-coital hours. Then there is the serotonin released during sex; this leaves you with that feeling of satiety and is proven to help reduce stress. Also calming are the endorphins, which are nature's weapon against pain and depression, and which Aveda founder Horst Rechelbacher calls "nature's beauty remedy." Add to that the fact that doing it with some zeal can get your heart rate nice and high, offering up all the same benefits as cardiovascular exercise. Maybe it's for all of these reasons that sex seems to slow the aging process.[12] Don't be glum, though, if you don't currently have a partner. Just make sure you're doing it solo, because orgasm alone is responsible for some of these perks.

A big plus to sharing the act is oxytocin, aka the love hormone: that's the thing that makes us cuddle after sex. The good news is that we don't *need* the intercourse to increase our levels. Basically any kind of warm, physical bonding, be it with friends or kids or even animals, can get the job done. Oxytocin has many of the same stress-lowering, happiness-inducing effects that we've already covered and also gives us the warm fuzzies, increasing both our sense of trust and empathy. Best of all, research seems to indicate that it has skin rejuvenating properties. *Now* we're talkin'. Rats with cuts injected with oxytocin healed twice as quickly as those who weren't injected.[13] It's also basically a natural diuretic, lowering the body's sodium content and reducing water retention.[14] Note to self: make love, not war, during PMS.

Given all the health and beauty benefits of sex and love, it's a small wonder that so many studies seem to indicate that married people are healthier.[15] Just a second, though. Don't be dialing some marriage-happy guy you dumped just yet. People love talking about these studies, but sometimes you have to dig below the surface to get to the truth of it—and to account for gender bias. It turns out that while *all* married men appear to be healthier than nonmarried ones—regardless of the quality of the union—when it comes to women, the benefits of matrimony exist only if she's happy. In fact, unhappily married women are the least healthy of the lot.[16] And for you single gals who find this whole marriage convo tedious, you can take pleasure in knowing that you ladies are the thinnest.

### Remember to Breathe

Regulating your breath may be the quickest and simplest way to improving your health. In his book *Breathing*, Dr. Andrew Weil says, "If I had to limit my advice on healthier living to just one tip, it would be simply to learn how to breathe correctly."[17]

And if you know anything about Weil, you know he's not messing around, because this guy has *a lot* of health advice. Simply bringing your attention to and deepening your breath can relax the mind and give the body necessary oxygen that we're not always getting, due to short or shallow breathing. That's a good starting point, and we already know that oxygenation and relaxation have their beauty benefits. If you want to take the practice further—and we think you should—there are many ways. We'll get more into some of those below.

### Enjoy Meditation and Other (Legal) Mind-Altering Techniques

Breathing exercises can be combined with mental and visual disciplines also known as meditation. While there are many different schools of practice, meditation usually involves stepping back from our relentless stream of thoughts and observing them as something separate from us. Then, once we get that part down, we find a place of inner calm. Of course, anyone who's tried knows that it's way easier said than done.

There are several very compelling studies on meditation's positive effects on brain patterns. One of those looks at a group of students, half of whom were given a mere five days of training in meditation. Not only did the novices outpace the control group in attention span, but also saliva tests showed reduced cortisol levels when given a stress-inducing math exam.[18] We thought that was pretty wild. Another study showed that more seasoned practitioners can control pain sensation, reducing it by up to 50 percent. During a tongue-piercing experiment, one meditator even exhibited a state of mind similar to that of someone on Quaaludes.[19] You just can't make this stuff up.

If you still think meditation is a bunch of new-age BS, take it from a dermatologist. Dr. Mostaghimi says, "Mindfulness meditation or cognitive behavioral therapy in addition to traditional treatments has shown to help clear the skin of patients with psoriasis and other skin conditions faster than traditional treatments alone." Put that in your pipe and smoke it.

There are other ways to slow down, if meditation isn't for you. We're both fans of acupuncture. It's helped us dramatically with certain ailments, like sciatica, chronic shoulder pain, and a bruised tailbone—not to mention anxiety and other emotional issues. (For the record: the needles are really, really small. And, no, they do not hurt. But for those still squeamish, there are variations that use vibrations and pressure instead.) Alexandra has also had amazing results with cranial sacral therapy, a subtle but almost magical type of treatment in the family of osteopathy.

Massages are great as well. Like all forms of enjoyable touch, they, too, can increase oxytocin levels.[20] So if you're not getting enough loving these days, booking a massage is a good idea. There's also some preliminary evidence that Reiki, a kind of nontouch energy treatment, is useful in reducing a variety of stress-related symptoms.[21] Call us flakes if you want, but even the most famous doctor in the world—Dr. Oz, obviously—has predicted that energy medicine will be the next big thing.

Regardless of the type of treatment you're into, there is one guaranteed benefit for all: actively making the choice to do something nice for yourself is a great way to show you that you love you. And that sort of self-care will have all kinds of positive effects on your life, and your face. If money's tight, there are great ways to supplement paid treatments (and we're going to tell you about one).

## BUTT OUT!
### It's Hard, but Not *That* Hard.

Just don't smoke. It's terrible for you. It's terrible for the people around you. And most of all, it is atrocious for your skin. It causes free-radical damage, dries and ages skin prematurely, delays wound healing, reduces blood flow to the skin,[22] can cause toxicity that presents itself in the form of lovely zit-like rashes (this has happened to us), causes upper-lip pucker wrinkles, turns your skin grey, and, perhaps you have heard, it also causes cancer. If that last thing isn't a good enough reason, maybe your mirror will be. According to a study from the Scripps Research Institute in California, smoking also increases glycation, a process that speeds up skin aging. (See the section on sugar in Chapter 9 for more on that evil process.) Another study by a plastic surgeon at Case Western Reserve University looked at identical twins who had aged differently. The study attempted to account for the nongenetic factors that altered the perceived age of the sisters, because obviously they had identical genes. Not surprisingly, smoking for ten years resulted in a perceived age at least two and a half years older than the nonsmoking twin.[23] (The other factors? Sun exposure, body mass index, and marital status.)

Acupuncture can stave off cravings, as can a host of other techniques. The patch and the gum have worked for lots of people we know, and if you can stick with it, then by all means, go cold turkey. Use whatever resources you need—there are plenty out there. This goes for the I-only-smoke-when-I-drink types, too. We know you. There are 19 million Americans, in fact, just like you: people who would probably tick the "no" box on the "Do you smoke?" line of a questionnaire. A recent study found that occasional smokers had a marked reduction in artery function for a week or longer after smoking. [24] There are also countless other studies that show the lasting impact of cigs in the system. These things don't leave our bodies with the last exhale. So if you smoke every Saturday night, well then, that's reduced function pretty much all the time. Convinced?

## DOING IT ALONE
### The Ayurvedic Art of Self-Massage

If you're looking for an affordable massage (such as a free one, say) and you don't have a boyfriend, lover, friend, or sister that you can nag, fear not. Ayurveda strongly encourages a daily self-massage ritual known as *abhyanga*. Sounds weird, but it's a wonderful way to start your day, and that's exactly what it's meant for. According to Ayurvedic texts—and no, we don't have any scientific studies here, just roll with it—the massage has numerous benefits. It's said to be both calming and energizing; to enhance circulation; to passify *vata* (which is the ADD-type energy that afflicts most everyone living in this century); and to help moisturize and nourish the skin. Regular practice is also said to release deep-seated toxins so that they can be eliminated. Apparently these ancient texts also say that *abhyanga* retards the aging process.

While we certainly can't endorse many of these claims, we'd sure like to believe them. It is definitely calming, and helps start the day off with clarity and a good dose of self love, so we don't really see a down side to incorporating it into your beauty and cleansing routine. Here's how you do it.

1. Choose an oil: unless you know your *dosha* or want to consult with an Ayurvedic doctor, you can just choose one of the recommended carrier oils like sesame, coconut, or almond.
2. Put it in a little plastic squeeze bottle.
3. Warm the bottle in hot water for about five minutes.
4. Either do this in the shower (but careful not to slip) or throw down a towel or mat that you don't mind ruining with oil. (Use the same one until it's too gross to bear and wash it on its own—do not put the oil-drenched towel in with the rest of your laundry.)
5. Work the warm oil over your entire body, starting at your feet.

6. Now, using strong up-and-down strokes over your limbs, and slightly lighter circular movements over your joints, midsection, and chest, massaging the oil into your skin. Give enough care to all of your parts; this process should take around ten minutes.

7. Take five minutes now to sit with your eyes closed and take deep, slow breaths.

8. Now take a shower, but use a really gentle cleanser (you don't want to strip away the healthy oil you've just so carefully applied).

---

## Why Yoga Will Make You Beautiful

We probably don't need to tell you about all the health and beauty benefits of yoga, but we're going to anyway. When this Indian practice first came west, it was just an oft-mocked offshoot of the hippie movement; now it's an oft-mocked mainstay of the health and fitness world, and we love it! About 16 million Americans practice yoga, and spending within the industry increased a whole 87 percent between 2004 and 2008 to a cool $6 billion dollars.[25]

If you're among the unconverted, read on. This single practice can pretty much kill a dozen birds with one hour-long workout. Here's how:

### Yoga and Other Sports

Yoga is proven to help prevent injuries by increasing flexibility and focus. That makes it a great supplemental workout for athletes and gym rats alike, so it's no wonder so many professional athletes have taken it up—like the Los Angeles Lakers, for instance. We hear they're pretty good.

### Yoga and Sleep

We know from personal experience that yoga helps us sleep better, but a recent study done at the University of Texas M.D. Anderson Cancer Center came to the same conclusion. Just twenty minutes of yoga a week seemed to help cancer patients fall asleep faster and sleep longer.[26]

### Yoga and Sex

Powerful thighs? Greater flexibility? Improved confidence? Yes, yes, and yes! All pretty obvious reasons why yoga may make sex better. But there's more: yoga enhances the mind's capacity to focus—not a bad thing in the sack. It also connects us to our bodies in a way that shows they are more than the sum of their parts. Certain postures also increase blood flow to the pelvis, generally a more constricted area, while others strengthen your Kegel muscles: two factors thought to make for better orgasms.[27]

### Yoga and Breath

Not to sound like the annoying yoga teacher, but yoga pretty much is about breathing. Even the most basic or beginner practice will teach you to focus on deeper inhalations and longer exhalations, and how to time them with your body's movement. Certain schools also teach more sophisticated techniques for breath work. There are entire books written on this stuff.

### Yoga and Toxins

It's a multipronged approach: between the twisting, the bending, the going upside down, and the breathing, you're actually massaging your organs, bringing more oxygen to the body, cir-

culating blood to undernourished areas, and ultimately improving lymphatic flow.[28] This makes yoga the ultimate in deep
detoxification. Oh, and you sweat. We've noticed that even in
slow classes we release lots of heat.

*Yoga and PMS*

According to yogis, regular practice can help with your hormones as well: standing on your head might help regulate your
pituitary gland; the peacock pose, your pancreas; and shoulder
stand, your thyroid.[29] Whatever the root, yoga appears to have
a positive impact on hormone balance, which is why we'd also
bet you dollars to donuts that regular yoga helps reduce your
PMS. (Careful, though: inversions and daily practice has also
been known to make your period kind of, um, hide. If you have
a light or irregular flow, take it easy when you're expecting
your monthly.)

*Yoga and Aging*

If you've ever been to a class before, you have almost certainly
heard this axiom: inversions, such as shoulder stands and
headstands, will keep you young. Why? By flipping you upside
down, inversions quite simply give your body a rest from the
downward pull. They also increase blood flow to the face
(good for skin) and to the heart, providing this mother-of-all
organs with some needed rest, all the while nourishing her with
fresh blood. It is commonly said that inversions have the same
benefits as rigorous exercise, minus all the panting. They're especially useful to people who spend a lot of time standing, or
who tend toward varicose veins, as well as other leg and circulation conditions.

## MAKE THE TIME

Feeling passionate about what you do is obviously ideal; but if you can't find it in your work, look for it elsewhere. If it's not exercise, maybe it's art, if it's not art, maybe it's horticulture. Whatever gets your juices juicing is what you need to make some time for. Along those lines, also just remember to create some space for yourself. That can mean any of the above activities (sleep doesn't count), or it can mean no activity at all. Turning off your phone, going someplace where nobody knows you, doing something that breaks from your routine can have an immediate positive effect on your outlook. And if you're gonna retain one thing from this chapter let it be this: your outlook is your look.

# Afterword

## Where We Go from Here

Horst Rechelbacher is the kind of guy who can and will talk for half an hour straight about different kinds of soil. His interest borders on obsession, and his knowledge is vast. When he's told you, almost breathlessly, why some fertilizers are better than others, he'll move on to greenhouse farming and plant chemistry and then, just to keep things interesting, he'll explain how it is that sex makes us beautiful.

What Rechelbacher doesn't talk a whole lot about is the beauty business, which is where he has made his fortune. It's also what he's spent the better portion of his life working at, from Aveda, which he founded in 1978, to Intelligent Nutrients, which he founded in 2008. During lunch, on the top floor of his two-story penthouse in downtown New York—a windowed sunroom full of angel busts—he walked us through his philosophy on leadership. Companies work best, he told us, when the head is connected to the body—Horst-speak for a high-level buy-in by a company's CEO. When he operated Aveda, he spent time visiting with suppliers, buyers, vendors, and store clerks—up and down the hierarchy—all the way to the lab. Rechelbacher isn't a chemist, but he studied and cared enormously about every single ingredient in his products.

Of course, he's a businessman, and a hugely successful one at that. Sometimes, he told us, that can get in the way of doing things how one thinks is best. "One gets romanced by the idea of business and profits," said Rechelbacher, recalling the decision to sell Aveda to Estée Lauder for $300 million. "I made some mistakes."

One of those mistakes, according to Rechelbacher, was being persuaded by a chemist that Aveda should expand into the hair dye market. "I didn't want to do hair color because I didn't think it was safe, [but a] chemist convinced me it could be safe, and I gave in. He also convinced me to use preservatives and phthalates, because they were 'safe,' too. There are still lots of people who claim that they are safe, especially at large companies, because they are effective. They work under all conditions to make the products stable—and a chemist's dream is that a product is stable. If it's not stable, he or she gets the heat. So the chemist makes it stable and says it is safe."

This is not an example of someone lazily ascribing blame. For a person with Rechelbacher's clout—whose success pivots on his expertise, and also on his name—to say he was misled tells us a lot about how dicey this business can be.

Rechelbacher says that when he sold his company to Estée Lauder, the products changed along with the leadership. "It's cost analysis first, and even with my products, they wanted to change everything to make the margins bigger. It's all about making profits, quick."

As we were finishing this book, Estée Lauder announced that its quarterly net sales were up 11 percent from the same period the previous year. During the worst recession in well over half a century, it saw $2.26 billion in net sales in just three months, showing once again just how robust and profitable the beauty industry is.[1]

When we took on this project, we had our own set of assumptions about how the industry operated. We found the vastness of the business daunting. We also assumed that the FDA must be on our side, and that despite its best intentions, it was powerless to safeguard us from the corporate cowboys trying to sell us expensive bottles of carcinogen-infused snake oil. We learned from Rechelbacher, however, and from everyone else we spoke to that it is not quite so easy to point the finger, and it's even harder to get straight answers.

When we asked Linda Katz, the head of the FDA's Office of Cosmetics and Colors, if she would like to see more power given to the FDA to regulate the beauty business, she said it doesn't matter what she thinks; it's up to Congress how much power her office is given. When we asked her to confirm her office's annual operating budget—reported to be a paltry $5.5 million—she said that was something she could not comment on. (This is not top-secret information; it's a government office.) When we asked her to characterize the FDA's relationship with the personal-care trade organization, she said she didn't understand the question. We were asking because the last guy who held her job now holds a prominent position at that industry group, which lobbies *against* cosmetics regulation. Her unwillingness to answer even the most softball questions confounded us.

People like to say that public officials answer to their constituents first, but if that's true, then why do activists' inquiries go unaddressed, as well as parents' complaints and journalists' questions? Why aren't we hearing more of a response to the growing rumble about these chemicals and the legitimate fears over our daily exposure to them? It's not just us talking; in fact, in certain circles, we probably seem a little late to the party. Ultimately, while the lawmakers aren't answering to us, they are most certainly answering to big business: they attend conferences, they sit in on meetings, they wine together and dine together, and they return each other's calls. But here's the clincher: with so little government oversight, it's not really the FDA that the beauty business answers to. It's us.

## BEACONS OF HOPE

Since we started researching this book, we've seen some momentum build on this subject. More journalists have tackled the topic, and the idea that our products might be unsafe has drifted slightly out of the hippie fringe—Dr. Oz has cautioned about unregulated and hazardous cosmetics, and Gisele launched her own, truly clean line. Naturally, we've also seen countless fake-natural brands hit the market—and a few legitimate, nontoxic ones as well. When it comes to the laws, however, we have a long way to go. Paving the way for national reform, however, is the state of California.

Back in 1986, California passed into law the Safe Drinking Water and Toxic Enforcement Act, or Proposition 65. The idea behind the law was simple: a business must not knowingly expose consumers to one of the seven hundred fifty or so chemicals listed in California as either carcinogens or reproductive toxicants without providing a "clear and reasonable warning."[2] On that list were many ingredients and contaminants—1,4-dioxane, toluene, lead, formaldehyde, and others[3]—that also end up in beauty products either by design or by accident. Until recently, little had been done to ensure that Prop 65 was also enforced for cosmetics.

Proposition 65 has established safe-harbor numbers for some three hundred chemicals—that means the law recognizes that in some cases, low levels of exposure are acceptable. In order to know if a cosmetics company is in violation of those levels, though, the state would need to know the actual amounts of chemicals used in the products—which is not data that's easy to come by.

It's not hopeless, though, especially when advocacy groups do some of the legwork to enforce the law. In 2008, following on the heels of an Organic Consumers Association (OCA) study, the California attorney general was able to mount a lawsuit against two companies whose body care products contained unsafe levels of the contaminant 1,4-dioxane: levels in violation of Prop 65.

California has made headway in other ways as well. In 2005, the state passed the California Safe Cosmetics Act. A kind of "right to know" law for consumers, the Cosmetics Act requires companies to report products that contain any of the chemicals on its list *regardless of levels used.* Expanding on the Prop 65 list—and based on criteria from the EPA, the National Toxicology Program, and the International Agency for Research on Cancer—the Cosmetics Act list features about eight hundred known carcinogens and reproductive and developmental toxicants. (Which are not quite the same as endocrine disruptors, but we were told that category is being discussed as a possible addition down the road.)

Dr. Michael DiBartolomeis, the toxicologist who heads up the program, says, "It purposely pushes something that is more of a precautionary approach, which means we don't care necessarily about the *levels* that are in there or whether they cause a theoretical risk. We care about whether the chemicals are in there period, and if they are, you have to tell us about it."

We have yet to see just how effective this program will be, but it does hold promise. For starters, it means those enforcing the laws will at least have a list of companies that are using banned ingredients. Second, there is a hope that by having to report the use of some of these heinous ingredients, manufacturers will be compelled to seek alternatives. It will also make it easy for the rest of us to find out if these chemicals of concern are used in some of our (old) favorite brands. It will be right there on a searchable website operated by California's public health department. This is obviously useful information to all of us— anything sold in California is probably also sold at a pharmacy near you. So this is a major step in the availability of user-friendly information about the dangerous ingredients in beauty products, and it will likely lead the way for other states, too.

As of this writing in early 2010, progress was underway in other parts of the country, as well. Minnesota followed California's lead toward stricter state regulation on cosmetics by banning all products that contain mercury as an intended ingredient.[4] It might seem like a small step, but we'll take it. It's also a big reminder to all of us to make some noise to our own state representatives because clearly some of them are listening. We can only hope that this growing attention will put the necessary pressure on companies to reformulate responsibly.

## HOW REAL CHANGE HAPPENS

While we applaud and support these efforts, the reality is that political progress is painfully slow. When it comes to effecting real change, the onus is on us. We think there are three simple ways to get that ball rolling.

The first way: well, you already did it. You learned something when you read this book, and we've learned something too. We encourage you to learn as much as you can: new reports come out all the time; new online resources; new books. Read whichever ones interest you the most. Find a natural beauty blog you love and bookmark it. If you think they all suck, start your own. Get to know Skin Deep and bookmark that, too. Keep tabs on the larger efforts to certify and clean up the natural market. Become an armchair expert. It's the best kind of expert to be: low-pressure, and you can do it with the TV on and dinner in your lap.

The second way: Tell your friends. Tell your mother. Tell your supervisor at work. Tell your kids. Tell your kids' teachers. Spread the word far and wide that until someone decides they have our back (we're looking at you, government), we're on our own. And while you're at it, tell Congress. Tell the FDA. And when you decide to switch your face cream, write the company you've abandoned, too.

Finally, and this is probably the most important part of all: the next time you go to the pharmacy to stock up on body lotion and shampoo, shaving cream and exfoliating scrub, pause. Pick up the bottle. Turn it upside down or backward. Read the ingredients list. If it's full of unhealthy ingredients—and it probably is—put it down. Vote with your wallet, and buy a clean product instead. Your body, and your looks, will thank you.

# Appendix A:
## The Ingredient Blacklist

Here's an alphabetized list of ingredients you don't want appearing on your labels. We've included it here for quick reference, but remember this: not all ingredients are created equal, so use that logical mind of yours. If several of these are showing up on a bottle, you can write off the brand with confidence. If just one appears on an otherwise clean list, then head to Skin Deep for a better picture, or call the company directly to ask them about it.

1,4-BENZENE (and variations like BENZENEDIAMINE, BENZENEDIOL etc.)

1,4-DIOXANE

ALUMINUM (including variations with CHLORIDE, HYDROCHLORIDE, CHLOROHYDRATE, HYDROXYBROMIDE, OXIDE, ZIRCONIUM etc.)

AMMONIUM LAURYL SULFATE

AMMONIUM PERSULFATE

BENZALKONIUM CHLORIDE

BORIC ACID (and several variations beginning with BOR)

BRONOPOL, aka 2-BROMO-2-NITROPROPANE-1,3-DIOL (with other variations)

BUTYLATED HYDROXYANISOLE (BHA)

BUTYLATED HYDROXYTOLUENE

BUTYLPARABEN

CETEARETH (including all number variations)

CHLOROACETAMIDE

COAL TAR

COCAMIDE DEA

COCAMIDE MEA

D&C RED 30 LAKE

D&C VIOLET 2

DEA OLETH-3 PHOSPHATE

DEA-CETYL PHOSPHATE

DIAZOLIDINYL UREA

DIBUTYL PHTHALATE

DIETHANOLAMINE (DEA)

DIHYDROXYBENZENE

DISODIUM EDTA

DMDM HYDANTOIN

ETHYLPARABEN

EUGENOL

FD&C DYES

FICUS CARICA or FIG EXTRACT

FORMALDEHYDE (including when
    followed by RESIN, SOLUTION,
    etc.)

FORMALIN

FORMIC ALDEHYDE

FRAGRANCE

HOMOSALATE

HYDROQUINONE

HYDROXYBENZOATE

HYDROXYBENZOIC ACID

HYDROXYPHENOL

IMIDAZOLIDINYL UREA

IODOPROPYNYL
    BUTYLCARBAMATE

ISOBUTYLPARABEN

LAURAMIDE DEA

LANOLIN

LAURETH-7

LEAD ACETATE

LECITHIN

LIGHT LIQUID PARAFFIN

MANGANESE SULFATE

METHYL ALDEHYDE

METHYLBENZENE

METHYLPARABEN

MINERAL OIL

MONOETHANOLAMINE (MEA)

MYRISTAMIDE DEA

NONOXYNOL

OCTINOXATE

OCTOXYNOL (usually followed by a
    number)

OCTYL-METHOXYCINNAMATE

OLEAMIDE DEA

OXYBENZONE

PABA

PADIMATE-O

PARAFFIN

PARFUM

PEG (followed by any number)

PERFUME

PETROLATUM

PETROLEUM DISTILLATE

PHENOL

PHENOXYETHANOL

PLACENTAL EXTRACT

POLYETHYLENE

POLYETHYLENE GLYCOL

POLYETHYLENE
    TEREPHTHALATE

POLYOXYETHYLENE

POLYSORBATE-80

POTASSIUM PERSULFATE

P-PHENYLENEDIAMINE

PROPYL ACETATE

PROPYLENE GLYCOL

PROPYLPARABEN

QUATERNIUM-15

RESORCINOL

SACCHARIN

SODIUM LAURETH SULFATE

SODIUM LAURYL SULFATE

SODIUM METABISULFATE

SODIUM METHYLPARABEN

STEARAMIDE MEA

STODDARD SOLVENT

TALC

TALCUM POWDER

TEFLON

TEA LAURYL SULFATE

TRETRASODIUM EDTA

THIMEROSAL

THIOGLYCOLIC ACID

TOLUENE

TRICLOSAN

TRIETHANOLAMINE

TRIPHENOLPHOSPHATE

# Appendix B:
# Resources

*The Body Toxic: How the Hazardous Chemistry of Everyday Things Threatens Our Health and Well-Being,* by Nena Baker (New York: North Point Press, 2009). A look at all consumer products and the toxics they expose us to, with a good chapter on personal care.

*Perfect Health: The Complete Mind/Body Guide,* by Deepak Chopra (Easton, PA: Harmony Press, 2001). Based on ancient Indian philosophy, Chopra outlines the keys to great health (which gives back as great beauty).

*Skinny Bitch: No-nonsense, Tough-love Guide for Savvy Girls Who Want to Stop Eating Crap And Start Looking Fabulous!,* by Rory Freedman and Kim Barnouin (Philadelphia, PA: Running Press, 2005). These spitfires launched a million vegan diets with their bestseller, which looked at how the evils of the food industry were impacting women's looks.

*The Green Beauty Guide: Your Essential Resource to Organic and Natural Skin Care, Hair Care, Makeup, and Fragrances,* by Julie Gabriel (Deerfield Beach, FL: HCI, 2008). The exhaustive eco-chick beauty book, with loads of recipes and research about skin care.

*The Truth About Beauty: Transform Your Looks and Your Life from the Inside Out,* by Kat James (New York: Atria Books, 2007). This is a great read for a more in-depth look at how beauty products, food, and wellness impact our looks and our health.

*Not Just a Pretty Face: The Ugly Side of the Beauty Industry*, by Stacy Malkan (Gabriola Island, British Columbia, Canada: New Society Publishers, 2007). The seminal book about toxics in beauty products, *Not Just a Pretty Face* is a great resource for those who want to know more.

*Cradle to Cradle: Remaking the Way We Make Things*, by William A. McDonough (New York: North Point Press, 2002). The seminal environmental book about products' life cycles, it isn't about beauty per se, but it gets you thinking about the impact of your actions.

*Women's Bodies Women's Wisdom: Creating Physical and Emotional Health and Healing*, by Christiane Northrup (New York: Bantam, 2006). Because you can't have good skin if you don't get to know and care for your body, we recommend the queen, Dr. Christiane Northrup.

*YOU: Being Beautiful: The Owner's Manual to Inner and Outer Beauty*, by Dr. Mehmet Oz and Michael F. Roizen (New York: Free Press, 2008). Dr. Oz and Roizen put you in control of your own body and beauty. It's an approach we like, and their recommendations seem to skew natural.

*The Omnivore's Dilemma: A Natural History of Four Meals*, Michael Pollan (New York: Penguin, 2007). Yet another book that helped further consumer understanding of where things come from, and how to make more conscientious choices.

*Absolute Beauty: Radiant Skin and Inner Harmony Through the Ancient Secrets of Ayurveda*, by Dr. Pratima Raichur (New York: Harper Paperbacks, 1999). The leading expert in Ayurvedic beauty techniques gives up recipes and tips for all skin types.

*Fast Food Nation*, by Eric Schlosser (New York: Harper Perennial, 2005). Because the food industry operates similarly to the beauty business, and because the more we know about both, the more thoughtful we become about our choices.

*Spontaneous Healing: How to Discover and Embrace Your Body's Natural Ability to Maintain and Heal Itself*, by Dr. Andrew Weil

(New York: Ballantine, 2000). We love Dr. Weil and think that, generally speaking, he gives out great advice about nutrition. This is our favorite, but you can't go wrong with any of his books.

*A Consumer's Dictionary of Cosmetics Ingredients: Complete Information About the Harmful and Desirable Ingredients Found in Cosmetics and Cosmeceuticals*, by Ruth Winter (New York: Three Rivers Press, 2005). This is a must-have reference book. Winter is middle of the road when it comes to toxics, and her research is exhaustive.

## FILMS WORTH WATCHING

*Good Hair.* Chris Rock's documentary focuses on black women's hair and the beauty industry that surrounds it. He even visits a science lab to learn about the awful chemicals in relaxers.

*Flow.* This film looks at the privatization of water and the increased concern over chemical contamination of our water sources.

*Food Inc.* If you don't see the connection between the food and cosmetics industry, you will after watching this.

## SHOPPING

**ABC Apothecary**. The New York City institution has dedicated a significant chunk of its first floor to nontoxic personal care. It skews high-end and fair-trade, with an emphasis on ecologically sound products.

**Beautorium.com**. This site carries a lot of brands other sites don't. We like the selection and the variety of things all in one place.

**BestInBeauty.com**. A natural beauty store site that's also proactive. They offer educational tools for readers and have worked to raise awareness about the industry through clever viral marketing campaigns.

**Evolue.com**. Finally, L.A. women have a place where they can touch, smell, try, and buy some of the best in clean beauty. Also offered are facials and mani-peds.

**Futurenatural.com**. This site carries all our favorite brands, looks great, and has free samples with every order.

**Saffronrouge.com**. A beauty site with classy, boutique, and affordable options, and it has a strcit list of criteria for what it'll carry.

**SpiritBeautyLounge.com**. We love this site. It's luxurious and pampery, with a good selection of carefully vetted (and attractive-looking) products. Free samples and a good return policy, too.

**Target**. Target gets a big high-five for a major chain pioneering into the naturals market. It carries some very reliable, high-quality brands we love at affordable prices.

**W3LL People**. A concept store with its own line of concentrated-pigment cosmetics, this is a chic, natural-beauty shop in Austin, Texas, started by a dermatologist, makeup artist, and environmentalist.

**Whole Foods**. Whole Foods does some of the work for you by carrying only brands that meet its Whole Body standards. Better for shampoos and body soaps than makeup, though.

**TheNatureofBeauty.com**. This site carries some fabulous European brands that are hard to find and are high-performance, and the criteria for getting on the site is strict. There is also a good selection of affordable options.

## LEARN MORE

**Cosmeticsdatabase.com**. This is the ultimate beauty and personal care database, founded by Stacy Malkan and the Campaign for Safe Cosmetics. It's a comprehensive searchable database of almost every product you can think of, with complete ingredient lists and information about all ingredients.

**EWG.org**. The Environmental Working Group, a watchdog organiation behind the Skindeep Database, has a great site with frequently updated information about ongoing studies, research, and lobbying efforts.

**PubMed.org**. This is a treasure trove of medical research about everything under the sun in mainstream medicine. It includes toxicological studies about ingredients of concern, skin care techniques and sometimes even alternative treatments.

## THINGS YOU CAN DO

Write to the FDA Office of Cosmetics and Colors, at (HFS-106) 5100 Paint Branch Parkway, College Park, MD, 20140, and give them a piece of your mind.

Write to members of Congress at Congress.org, to tell them you want to see more oversight granted to the FDA.

Team up with a local chapter of Teens Turning Green. Find them at teensturninggreen.org.

When you change your product, write the company a letter telling them you have, and then blog it, tweet it, and change your status update on Facebook.

Give this book to your mother and your sister and your best friend.

# Notes

## CHAPTER 1. WHY WE'RE COMING CLEAN

1. "Health Alarm over New Hair Straightener: BKT, Treatment from Brazil, Contains Known Cancer-Causer," October 26, 2007. http://www.cbsnews.com/stories/2007/10/26/earlyshow/health/main3414868.shtml.

2. Halina Szeinwald Brown, Donna R. Bishop, and Carol A. Rowan, "The Role of Skin Absorption as a Route of Exposure for Volatile Organic Compounds (VOCs) in Drinking Water," *American Journal of Public Health*, May 1984, 74 (5): 479–484.

3. Stacy Malkan, *Not Just a Pretty Face* (Gabriola Island: New Society Publishers, 2007).

4. Companies offering newer versions of this kind of procedure claim to have eliminated formaldehyde from their formulas, but because it is uncommon for salons to share complete ingredient lists with their clients, we remain skeptical.

## CHAPTER 2. THE REGULATION GAME

1. Madeleine Bird, "Toxins in Toiletries," http://www.cwhn.ca/fr/node/39367.

2. "Amyl Cinnamal: What Is It?" http://www.cosmeticsinfo.org/ingredient_details.php?ingredient_id=1914.

3. Amy Marsh, "Toxic Chemicals Found in Designer Fragrance: Environmental Health Network Petitions FDA to Have Eternity Misbranded," May 1999, http://www.snowcrest.net/lassen/eiehn03.html.

4. Ibid. "Analysis Summary: Calvin Klein's Eternity eau de parfum," http://users.lmi.net/~wilworks/FDApetition/analysis.htm.

5. Ibid.

6. "Food and Drugs: Requirements for Specific Cosmetic Products," http://ecfr.gpoaccess.gov/cgi/t/text/text-idx?c=ecfr;rgn=div6;view=text;node=21%3A7.0.1.2.10.2;idno=21;sid=11932eedf179169919a4f92bf2ebd207;cc=ecfr.

7. "FDA Authority over Cosmetics: What Does the Law Say About Cosmetic Safety and Labeling?," March 3, 2005, http://www.fda.gov/Cosmetics/Guidance ComplianceRegulatoryInformation/ucm074162.htm.

8. Ibid.

9. "Significant Dates in U.S. Food and Drug Law History," http://www.fda. gov/AboutFDA/WhatWeDo/History/Milestones/ucm128305.htm.

10. "Federal Food and Drugs Act of 1906," http://www.fda.gov/Regulatory Information/Legislation/ucm148690.htm#sec1.

11. A. F. Kantor. "Upton Sinclair and the Pure Food and Drugs Act of 1906: 'I Aimed at the Public's Heart and By Accident I Hit It in the Stomach,'" December 1976.

12. Teresa Riordan, *Inventing Beauty: A History of the Innovations that Have Made Us Beautiful* (New York: Broadway, 2004).

13. "Concealing the Truth: The Hidden Dangers of Makeup," http://www. faculty.virginia.edu/metals/cases/sheehan3.html.

14. Riordan, *Inventing Beauty.*

15. R. C. Jamieson, "Eyelash Dye (Lash-Lure) Dermatitis with Conjunctivitis," *Journal of the American Medical Association*, 1933, 101 (2): 1560.

16. "FDA Authority over Cosmetics."

17. "Significant Dates in U.S. Food and Drug Law History."

18. Ibid.

19. "Personal Care Products Council History," http://www.personalcare council.org/Content/NavigationMenu/About_Us/History/History_3.htm.

20. Norman F. Estrin and James M. Akerson, eds., *Cosmetic Regulation in a Competitive Environment* (London: Informa Health Care, 2000).

21. "Cosmeceutical," February 24, 2000, http://www.fda.gov/Cosmetics/ ProductandIngredientSafety/ProductInformation/ucm127064.htm.

22. *Personal Care Products Council 2008 Annual Report*, Washington, DC.

23. Nena Baker, *The Body Toxic: How the Hazardous Chemistry of Everyday Things Threatens Our Health and Well-being* (San Francisco, CA: North Point Press, 2009), 92; and Ruth Winter, *A Consumer's Dictionary of Cosmetics Ingredients: Complete Information About the Harmful and Desirable Ingredients Found in Cosmetics and Cosmeceuticals* (New York: Three Rivers Press, 2005).

24. "About the Personal Care Products Council," http://www.personalcare council.org/Template.cfm?Section=About_Us.

25. *Personal Care Products Council 2008 Annual Report*, C8.

26. "A Centennial History of the Personal Care Products Council: Highlights

of the Council's Role in the Personal Care Products Industry for More Than 100 Years," http://www.personalcarecouncil.org/Content/NavigationMenu/About_Us/History/History.htm.

27. *Personal Care Products Council 2008 Annual Report*, C11.

28. Ibid.

29. "CIR Panel and Staff," http://www.cir-safety.org/panelandstaff.shtml.

30. Cosmetic Ingredient Review homepage, http://www.cir-safety.org/.

31. Cosmetic Ingredient Review Expert Panel Meeting, March 23–24, 2009, meeting minutes.

32. "FDA Fails to Protect Consumers: Consumer Update—FDA Admits Inability to Ensure the Safety of Personal Care Products," October 5, 2005, http://www.cosmeticsdatabase.com/research/fdafails.php.

33. *Personal Care Products Council 2008 Annual Report*, C18.

34. Kia Franklin, "Kerry Says: Don't Shut Consumers Out of Product Safety Conference," September 27, 2007, http://www.tortdeform.com/archives/2007/09/kerry_says_dont_shut_consumers_1.html.

35. Bird, "Toxins in Toiletries."

36. According to Dr. Ladd Smith at RIFM, interviewed by authors August 9, 2009.

37. "About Us," http://www.rifm.org/about.asp.

38. "Fragrance: What Is It?" http://www.cosmeticsinfo.org/ingredient_details.php?ingredient_id=1420.

39. "IFRA Code of Practice," October 2006, http://www.ifraorg.org/Home/Code,%20Standards%20Compliance/Code-of-Practice/page.aspx/88 (from the PDF).

40. P. S. Spencer, A. B. Sterman, D. S. Horoupian, and M. M. Foulds, "Neurotoxic Fragrance Produces Ceroid and Myelin Disease," May 11, 1979, 204 (4394): 633–635.

## CHAPTER 3. DIRTY INGREDIENTS

1. "EWG Research Shows 22 Percent of All Cosmetics May Be Contaminated with Cancer-Causing Impurity," Environmental Working Group News Release, February 8, 2007, http://www.ewg.org/node/21286.

2. "A Little Prettier," Campaign for Safe Cosmetics Report, December 18, 2008, http://www.ewg.org/report/toxic-tub/31209.

3. Ibid.

4. "1,4-Dioxane," U.S. Environmental Protection Agency, http://www.epa.gov/ttnatw01/hlthef/dioxane.html.

5. "Public Health Statement for 1,4-Dioxane," Agency for Toxic Substances

& Disease Registry, September 2007, http://www.atsdr.cdc.gov/toxprofiles/phs187.html.

6. http://www.fda.gov/Cosmetics/ProductandIngredientSafety/Potential-Contaminants/ucm101566.htm; and "Public Health Statement for 1,4-Dioxane," Agency for Toxic Substances & Disease Registry, http://www.atsdr.cdc.gov/toxprofiles/phs187.html.

7. Campaign for Safe Cosmetics Press Release, "Cancer-Causing Chemical Found in Children's Bath Products," February 8, 2007, http://www.safecosmetics.org/article.php?id=64.

8. B. P. He and M. J. Strong, "A-Morphological Analysis of the Motor Neuron Degeneration and Microglial Reaction in Acute and Chronic in Vivo Aluminum Chloride Neurotoxicity," *Journal of Chemical Neuroanatomy*, January 2000, 17 (4): 207–215.

9. Philippa D. Darbre, "Aluminium, Antiperspirants, and Breast Cancer." *Journal of Inorganic Biochemistry*, September 2005, 99 (9): 1912–1919.

10. Christopher Exley, Lisa M. Charles, Lester Barr, Claire Martin, Anthony Polwart, and Philippa D. Darbre, "Aluminium in Human Breast Tissue," *Journal of Inorganic Biochemistry*, September 2007, 101 (9): 1344–1346.

11. Ibid.

12. Kim Painter, "Sun Dangers Spelled Out in UVA, UVB, SPF," USAToday.com, May 7, 2007.

13. M. Coronado, H. De Haro, X. Deng, M. A. Rempel, R. Lavado, and D. Schlenk, "Estrogenic Activity and Reproductive Effects of the UV-filter Oxybenzone (2-hydroxy-4-methoxyphenyl-methanone) in Fish," *Aquatic Toxicology*, November 21, 2008, 90 (3): 182–187; and "Summer 2009 Sees Dramatic Shift in Sunscreen Industry," Environmental Working Group, http://www.ewg.org/cosmetics/report/sunscreen09/investigation/summary-of-findings.

14. Molly Raunch, "Blocking Sun," http://www.thegreenguide.com/personal-care/blocking-sun.

15. "Coal Tar," Cosmetics Database, http://www.cosmeticsdatabase.com/ingredient.php?ingred06=701514.

16. Catherine Zandonella, "The Dirty Dozen Chemicals in Cosmetics, September 18, 2007, http://www.thegreenguide.com/personal-care/dirty-dozen.

17. Judith H. J. Roelofzen, Katja K. H. Aben, Pieter G. M. van der Valk, Jeanete L. M. van Houtum, Peter C. M. van de kerkhof, L. A. Kiemeney, "Coal Tar in Dermatology," *Journal of Dermatological Treatment*, 2007, 18(6): 329–334.

18. "Diethanolamine," U.S. Food and Drug Administration, fda.gov, October 27, 2001.

19. "Cocamide Dea," Cosmetics Database, http://www.cosmeticsdatabase.com/ingredient/701516/COCAMIDE_DEA/.

20. "Toxicology and Carcinogenesis Studies of Coconut Oil Acid Diethanolamine Condensate (CAS No. 68603-42-9) in F344/N Rats and B6C3F1 Mice (Dermal Studies)," *National Toxicology Program Technical Report Series*, January 2001, 479: 5–226.

21. "Diethanolamine," fda.gov.

22. Michael S. Roberts and Kenneth A. Walthers, *Dermal Absorption and Toxicity Assessment* (New York: Informa Health Care, 1998).

23. "Study Shows Ingredient Commonly Found in Shampoos May Inhibit Brain Development," August 3, 2006, *ScienceDaily*, http://www.sciencedaily.com/releases/2006/08/060803182218.htm.

24. http://monographs.iarc.fr/ENG/Monographs/vol88/mono88.pdf.

25. "Formaldehyde," http://www.cosmeticsdatabase.com/ingredient.php?ingred06=702500.

26. Alexandra Drosu, "Brazilian Hair Straighteners Offer Reformulated Keratin Treatments," *Los Angeles Times*, August 17, 2008.

27. "Final Report on Carcinogens Background for Formaldehyde," National Toxicology Program, U.S. Department of Health and Human Services, January 22, 2010.

28. P. S. Spencer, M. C. Bischoff-Fenton, O. M. Moreno, D. L. Opdyke, and R. A. Ford, "Neurotoxic Properties of Musk Ambrette," *Toxicology and Applied Pharmacology*, September 30, 1985, 75 (3): 571–575; and S. M. Caress and A. C. Steinemann, "Prevalence of Fragrance Sensitivity in the American Population," *Journal of Environmental Health*, March 2009, 71 (7): 46–50.

29. Thomas Fuller, "Glamour at a Price in Asia—Health & Science—International Herald Tribune," *New York Times*, May 1, 2006.

30. Winter, *A Consumer's Dictionary of Cosmetics Ingredients*, 294.

31. Ibid.

32. http://futurederm.com/2007/10/18/spotlight-on-hydroquinone/.

33. Winter, *A Consumer's Dictionary of Cosmetics Ingredients*, 294.

34. Guy Montague-Jones, "Minnesota Bans Mercury from Cosmetics," January 2, 2008, http://www.cos\meticsdesign.com/Formulation-Science/Minnesota-bans-mercury-from-cosmetics.

35. "FDA Study: Lead Levels in Lipstick Much Higher Than Previously Reported," Campaign for Safe Cosmetics Press Release, September 1, 2009, http://www.reuters.com/article/pressRelease/idUS170678+01-Sep-2009+PRN20090901.

36. E. Katz, R. Lovel, W. Mee, and F. Solomon, "Citizens' Panel on Nanotechnology Report to Participants," April 2005, http://www.minerals.csiro.au/sd/pubs/Citizens_Panel_Report_to_Participants_April_2005_final_110.pdf;

and S. Allen Counter, "Whitening Skin Can Be Deadly," Boston.com News, December 16, 2003, http://www.boston.com/news/globe/health_science/articles/2003/12/16/whitening_skin_can_be_deadly/.

37. Steven Marcus, "Toxicity, Lead," August 2009, http://emedicine.medscape.com/article/815399-overview.

38. Barry M. Diner, "Toxicity, Mercury," September 18, 2009, http://emedicine.medscape.com.

39. "Analysis," Project on Emerging Nanotechnologies, http://www.nanotechproject.org/inventories/consumer/analysis_draft/.

40. "Consumer Products Inventory," Project on Emerging Nanotechnologies, http://www.nanotechproject.org/inventories/consumer/search/page6/?search=1&country_origin=4586&categories=4528&subcategories=4556.

41. "EU Regulates Use of Nano Particles in Cosmetics," July 16, 2009, http://www.earthtimes.org/articles/show/277669,eu-regulates-use-of-nano-particles-in-cosmetics.html.

42. Sheryl Ubelacker, "Heading to Medicine from Science Fiction," *Globe and Mail*, January 8, 2009, http://www.theglobeandmail.com/news/technology/science/heading-to-medicine-from-science-fiction/article964161/.

43. Winter, *A Consumer's Dictionary of Cosmetics Ingredients*, 32.

44. Osamu Handa, Satoshi Kokura, Satoko Adachi, Tomohisa Takagi, Yuji Naito, Toru Tanigawa, Norimasa Yoshida, and Toshikazu Yoshikawa, "Methylparaben Potentiates UV-induced Damage of Skin Keratinocytes," *Toxicology*, October 2006, 227 (1–2): 62–72; and Simon Pitman, "Aging Claims Put Parabens Back under the Spotlight," August 25, 2005, http://www.cosmeticsdesign-europe.com/FormulationScience/Ageing-claims-put-parabens-back-under-the-spotlight.

45. Leslie S. Baumann, "Parabens. (Cosmeceutical Critique)," October 2007, http://www.entrepreneur.com/tradejournals/article/170017582.html.

46. P. W. Harvey and P. Darbre, "Endocrine Disrupters and Human Health: Could Oestrogenic Chemicals in Body Care Cosmetics Adversely Affect Breast Cancer Incidence in Women?" *Journal of Applied Toxicology*, May–June 2004, 24 (3): 167–176.

47. Dawn M., "Petrochemical Compounds: An Introduction," February 9, 2009, http://toxicbeauty.co.uk/blog/2009/02/09/petrochemical-compounds-an-introduction/; and "Petroleum Distillates," *Cosmetics Info*, http://www.cosmeticsinfo.org/ingredient_details.php?ingredient_id=891.

48. "EPA Comments on Chemical RTK HPV Challenge Submission: Petroleum Oxidates and Derivatives Thereof Category, March 27, 2003.

49. J. V. Lacey Jr., D. H. Garabrant, T. J. Laing, B. W. Gillespie, M. D. Mayes,

B. C. Cooper, and D. Schottenfeld, "Petroleum Distillate Solvents as Risk Factors for Undifferentiated Connective Tissue Disease (UCTD)," *American Journal of Epidemiology*, April 15, 1999, 149 (8): 761–770.

50. Bernard A. Hildebrand Jr., "Undifferentiated Connective-Tissue Disease," July 24, 2009, http://emedicine.medscape.com/article/334482-overview.

51. "Household Products Containing Petroleum Distillates and Other Hydrocarbons; Advance Notice of Proposed Rulemaking; Extension of Comment Period," U.S. Environmental Protection Agency, April 28, 1997.

52. Dawn M., "Petrochemical Compounds."

53. "Household Products Containing Petroleum Distillates and Other Hydrocarbons."

54. M. Sir Hashim, Y. O. Hamza, B. Yahia, F. M. Khogali, and G. I. Sulieman, "Poisoning from Henna Dye and Para-phenylenediamine Mixtures in Children in Khartoum," *Annals of Tropical Paedriatrics*, 1992, 12 (1): 3–6.

55. Winter, *A Consumer's Dictionary of Cosmetics Ingredients*, 402.

56. Y. C. Huang, W. C. Hung, W. Y. Kang, W. T. Chen, and C. Y. Chai, "P-Phenylenediamine Induced DNA Damage in SV-40 Immortalized Human Uroepithelial Cells and Expression of Mutant P53 and COX-2 Proteins," *Toxicology Letters*, April 2007, 170 (2): 116–123.

57. E. Lee, S. An, D. Choi, S. Moon, and I. Chang, "Comparison of Objective and Sensory Skin Irritations of Several Cosmetic Preservatives." *Contact Dermatitis*, March 2007, 56 (3): 131–136.

58. James C. Lamb, Jerry R. Reel, A. Davis Lawton, and Donald B. Feldman, "Reproductive Toxicology: Ethylene Glycol Moonophenyl Ether," *Environmental Health Perspectives*, February 1997, 105 (1): 225–226.

59. "Final Report on the Safety Assessment of Phenozyethanol," *International Journal of Toxicology*, 1990, 9 (2): 259–277.

60. "Mommy's Bliss Nipple Cream," U.S. Food and Drug Administration Safety Information, http://www.fda.gov/Safety/MedWatch/SafetyInformation/SafetyAlertsforHumanMedicalProducts/ucm092727.htm.

61. Ibid.

62. "Pthalates," Human Toxome Project at Environmental Working Group, http://www.ewg.org/sites/humantoxome/chemicals/chemical_classes.php?class=Phthalate.s

63. "A Little Prettier," Campaign for Safe Cosmetics Report, http://www.safecosmetics.org/downloads/A-Little-Prettier_Dec08.pdf.

64. Evanthia Diamanti-Kandarakis, Jean-Pierre Bourguignon, Linda C. Giudice, Russ Hauser, Gail S. Prins, Ana M. Soto, R. Thomas Zoeller, and Andrea C. Gore, "Endocrine-Disrupting Chemicals," *Endocrine Society Report*, 2009.

65. H. Ohtani, I. Miura, and Y. Ichikawa, "Effects of Dibutyl Phthalate as an Environmental Endocrine Disruptor on Gonadal Sex Differentiation of

Genetic Males of the Frog Rana Rugosa," *Environmental Health Perspective*, December 2000, 108 (12): 1189–1193.

66. "Formaldehyde, 2-Butoxuethanol and 1-tert-Butoxypropan-2-ol; Summary of Data Reported and Evaluation," World Health Organization's International Agency for Research on Cancer, December 2006, http://monographs. iarc.fr/ENG/Monographs/vol88/volume88.pdf.

67. "Propylene Glycol," International Programme on Chemical Safety Poisons Information, Monograph 443, http://www.inchem.org/documents/pims/chemical/pim443.htm#SectionTitle:5.3%20%20Dermal.

68. "Formaldehyde," Cosmetics Database, http://www.cosmeticsdatabase. com/ingredient.php?ingred06=702500#.

69. R. S. Laniga and T. A. Yamarik, "Final Report on the Safety Assessment of PEG-6, -8, and -20 Sorbitan Beeswax," *International Journal of Toxicology*, 2001, 20 (4): 27–38.

70. L. Chahine, N. Sempson, and C. Wagoner, "The Effect of Sodium Lauryl Sulfate on Recurrent Aphthous Ulcers: A Clinical Study." *Compend Contin Educ Dent*, December 1997, 18 (12): 1238–1240.

71. Roderick E. Black, Fred J. Hurley, and Donald C. Havery, "Occurrence of 1,4-Dioxane in Cosmetic Raw Materials and Finished Cosmetic Products," *Journal of AOAC International*, May 2001, 84 (3): 666–670.

72. B. L. Harlow, D. W. Cramer, and D. A. Bell, "Perineal Exposure to Talc and Ovarian Cancer Risk," *Obstetrics and Gynecology*, 1991, 80 (1): 19–26.

73. J. E. Muscat and M. S. Huncharek, "Perineal Talc Use and Ovarian Cancer: A Critical Review," *European Journal of Cancer Prevention*, April 2008, 17 (2): 139–146.

74. "Talcum Powder and Cancer," American Cancer Society, http://www. cancer.org/docroot/cri/content/cri_2_6x_talcum_powder_and_cancer.asp.

75. M. A. Gates, S. S. Tworoger, K. L. Terry, L. Titus-Ernstoff, B. Rosner, I. De Vivo, D. W. Cramer, and S. E. Hankinson, "Talc Use, Variants of the GSTM1, GSTT1, and NAT2 Genes, and Risk of Epithelial Ovarian Cancer," *Cancer Epidemiology, Biomarkers & Prevention: A Publication of the American Association for Cancer Research*, September 2008, 17 (9): 2436–2444.

76. Tana Kim, "Toluene," http://74.125.47.132/search?q=cache:4W-1uLLXz 80J: www.merit.uiuc.edu/documents/THERM_01.doc+coca-cola+toluene&cd =9&hl=en&ct=clnk&gl=us&client=firefox-a.

77. Lance A. Wallace, *Identification of Polar Volatile Organic Compounds in Consumer Products and Common Microenvironments*, U.S. Environmental Protection Agency Report, March 1, 1991, http://www.ourlittleplace.com/ epa.html; and "Toluene," The Good Scents Company, http://www.thegood scentscompany.com/data/rw1290031.html.

78. Winter, *A Consumer's Dictionary of Cosmetics Ingredients*, 102.

79. T. P. Ng, S. C. Foo, and T. Yoong, "Risk of Spontaneous Abortion in Workers Exposed to Toluene," *British Journal of Industrial Medicine*, November 1992, 49 (11): 804–807.

80. Ibid.

81. Aviva Glaser, "The Ubiquitous Triclosan; A Common Antibacterial Agent Exposed, Pesticides and You," 2004, 24 (3): 12–17, http://www.beyond pesticides.org/pesticides/factsheets/Triclosan%20cited.pdf.

82. Christie Bailey, "Triclosan Causes Antimicrobial Resistance," October 5, 2009, http://healthfieldmedicare.suite101.com/article.cfm/triclosan_causes_antimicrobial_resistance.

83. "Triclosan," European Commission: Health & Consumer Protection Directorate-General, October 10, 2006, http://ec.europa.eu/health/ph_risk/committees/04_sccp/docs/sccp_o_073.pdf.

84. Laura M. McMurry, Margret Oethinger, and Stuart B. Levy, "Triclosan Targets Lipid Synthesis," *Nature*, August 6, 1998, 394: 531–532.

85. Leah M. Zorrilla, Emily K. Gibson, Susan C. Jeffay, Kevin M. Crofton, Woodrow R. Setzer, Ralph L. Cooper, and Tammy E. Stoker, "The Effects of Triclosan on Puberty and Thyroid Hormones in Male Wistar Rats," *Toxicological Sciences*, October 21, 2008 107 (1): 56–64; and N. Veldhoen, R. C. Skirrow, H. Osachoff, H. Wigmore, D. J. Clapson, M. P. Gunderson, G. Van Aggelen, and C. C. Helbing, "The Bactericidal Agent Triclosan Modulates Thyroid Hormone-Associated Gene Expression and Disrupts Postembryonic Anuran Development," *Aquatic Toxicology*, December 1, 2006, 80 (3): 217–227.

86. Veldhoen et al., "The Bactericidal Agent Triclosan."

87. "Decoding the Cosmetic Label," U.S. Food and Drug Administration, February 3, 1995, *FDA Consumer*, http://www.ourlittleplace.com/label.html.

88. "Cosmetic Labeling Guide," Food and Drug Administration, October 1991, http://www.fda.gov/Cosmetics/CosmeticLabelingLabelClaims/CosmeticLabelingManual/ucm126444.htm#clgl3.

89. "Lotions and Potions," AARP, March 1, 2007, http://www.aarp.org/health/conditions/articles/harvard__skin-care-and-repair_6.html.

## CHAPTER 4. YOUR HAIR

1. Julie Gabriel, *The Green Beauty Guide: Your Essential Resource to Organic and Natural Skin Care, Hair Care, Makeup, and Fragrances* (Deerfield Beach, FL: HCI Books, 2008).

2. Winter, *A Consumer's Dictionary of Cosmetics Ingredients*, 455.

3. Gabriel, *The Green Beauty Guide*, 14.

4. Winter, *A Consumer's Dictionary of Cosmetics Ingredients*, 160.

5. "Monograph on the Evaluation of the Carcinogenic Risk of Chemicals to Humans: Some N-Nitroso Compounds," International Agency for Research on Cancer, 1978, 17: 77–82.

6. Mehmet Oz and Michael F. Roizen. *YOU: Being Beautiful: The Owner's Manual to Inner and Outer Beauty* (NY: Free Press, 2008), 80.

7. "Cancer in a Can: What the Chemical Industry Kept Secret About Vinyl Chloride in Hair Spray," Environmental Working Group, Chemical Industry Archives, http://www.chemicalindustryarchives.org/dirtysecrets/hairspray/1.asp.

8. Ibid.

9. G. Ormond, M. J. Nieuwenhuijsen, P. Nelson, M. B. Toledano, N. Iszatt, S. Geneletti, et al., "Endocrine Disruptors in the Workplace, Hair Spray, Folate Supplementation, and Risk of Hypospadias: Case–Control Study," *Environmental Health Perspectives*, November 2008.

10. Oz and Roizen, *YOU: Being Beautiful*, 71.

11. Ibid., 72.

12. K. Mochida, K. Ito, H. Harino, A. Kakuno, K. Fujii, "Acute Toxicity of Pyrithione Antifouling Biocides and Joint Toxicity with Copper to Red Sea Bream (Pagrus major) and Toy Shrimp (Heptacarpus futilirostris)," *Environmental Toxicology & Chemistry*, November 2006, 25 (11): 3058–3064; and S. D. Lamore, C. M. Cabello, G. T. Wondrak, "The Topical Antimicrobial Zinc Pyrithione Is a Heat Shock Response Inducer that Causes DNA Damage and PARP-Dependent Energy Crisis in Human Skin Cells," *Cell Stress Chaperones*, October 2009, http://www.ncbi.nlm.nih.gov/pubmed/19809895?ordinalpos=1&itool=EntrezSystem2.PEntrez.Pubmed.Pubmed_ResultsPanel.Pubmed_DefaultReportPanel.Pubmed_RVDocSum.

13. Andrew Weil, "Seeking Natural Psoriasis Relief?" http://www.drweil.com/drw/u/QAA400309/seeking-natural-psoriasis-relief.

14. George Kuepper, Raeven Thomas, and Richard Earles, "Use of Baking Soda as a Fungicide," *National Sustainable Agriculture Information Service*, November 2001.

15. Andrew Weil, "Six Tips for Healthy Hair and Skin," http://www.drweil.com/drw/u/ART02032/healhty-hair-and-skin.html.

16. Winter, *A Consumer's Dictionary of Cosmetics Ingredients*, 274.

17. Ibid., 396.

## CHAPTER 5. YOUR FACE

1. "Salicylic Acid," http://www.inchem.org/documents/pims/pharm/pim642.htm#SectionTitle:7.2%20%20Toxicity.

2. Paula Begoun, "Benzoyl Peroxide," Cosmetic Ingredient Dictionary, http://www.cosmeticscop.com/ingredient_dictionary.aspx?lid=498.

3. T. J. Slaga, A. J. Klein-Szanto, L. L. Triplett, L. P. Yotti, and K. E. Trosko, "Skin Tumor-Promoting Activity of Benzoyl Peroxide, A Widely Used Free Radical–Generating Compound," *Science*, August 28, 1981, 213 (4511): 1023–1025.

4. "Exploxive/Peroxidizable Chemicals," http://www.cheminfonet.org/explod.htm.

5. D. Flaxman and P. Griffiths, "Is Tea Tree Oil Effective at Eradicating MRSA Colonization? A Review," *British Journal of Community Nursing*, March 2005, 10 (3): 123–126.

6. I. B. Bassett, D. L. Pannowitz, and R. S. Barnetson, "A Comparative Study of Tea-Tree Oil Versus Benzoyl Peroxide in the Treatment of Acne," *Medical Journal of Australia*, October 15, 1990, 153 (8): 455–458.

7. Paula Begoun, "Salicylic Acid," *Cosmetic Ingredient Dictionary*, http://www.cosmeticscop.com/ingredient_dictionary.aspx?lid=532.

8. F. Di Renzo, G. Cappelletti, M. L. Broccia, E. Giavini, and E. Menegola, "The Inhibition of Embryonic Histone Deacetylases as the Possible Mechanism Accounting for Axial Skeletal Malformations Induced by Sodium Salicylate," *Toxicological Sciences*, August 2008, 104 (2): 397–404.

9. Anton C. de Groot, Johan Pieter Nater, and J. Willem Weyland, *Unwanted Effects of Cosmetics and Drugs Used in Dermatology* (Maryland Heights, MO: Elsevier, 1994), 260.

10. "Alpha Hydroxy Acids, http://www.webmd.com/vitamins-supplements/ingredientmono-977-ALPHA+HYDROXY+ACIDS.aspx?activeIngredientId=977&activeIngredientName=ALPHA+HYDROXY+ACIDS&source=2.

11. Paula Begoun, "AHAs," *Cosmetic Ingredient Dictionary*, http://www.cosmeticscop.com/dictionary_term.aspx?tid=757&lid=492&term=AHA.

12. http://www.fda.gov/Cosmetics/ProductandIngredientSafety/SelectedCosmeticIngredients/ucm107940.htm#q5.

13. "Has FDA Conducted Research on the Safety of AHAs?" http://www.ncbi.nlm.nih.gov/pubmed/12113844?dopt=Abstract; and "Alpha Hydroxy Acids," http://www.webmd.com/vitamins-supplements/ingredientmono-977-ALPHA+HYDROXY+ACIDS.aspx?activeIngredientId=977&activeIngredientName=ALPHA+HYDROXY+ACIDS&source=2.

14. "Guidance: Labeling for Cosmetics Containing Acids," January 10, 2005, http://www.fda.gov/Cosmetics/GuidanceComplianceRegulatoryInformation/GuidanceDocuments/ucm090816.htm.

15. Ibid.

16. G. B. Jemec and R. Na, "Hydration and Plasticity Following Long-Term

Use of a Moisturizer: A Single-blind Study," in *Acta Derm Venereol*, 2002, 82 (5): 322–324.

17. A. Budiyanto, N. U. Ahmed, A. Wu, T. Bito, O. Nikaido, T. Osawa, M. Ueda, and M. Ichihashi, "Protective Effect of Topically Applied Olive Oil Against Photocarcinogenesis Following UVB Exposure of Mice," *Carcinogenesis*, November 2000, 21 (11): 2085–2090.

18. C. Letawe, M. Boone, and G. E. Pierard. "Digital Image Analysis of the Effect of Topically Applied Linoleic Acid on Acne Microcomedones." *Clinical & Experimental Dermatology*, March 1998, 23 (2): 56–58.

19. H. Dobrev, "Clinical and Instrumental Study of the Efficacy of a New Sebum Control Cream," *Journal of Cosmetic Dermatology*, June 2007, 6 (2): 113–118.

20. "Oxybenzone," http://www.caslab.com/Oxybenzone.php5.

21. Hannah Morrison, "Botox Boom Among Young Women," *Newsbeat*, February 26, 2008.

22. Dr. Oz and Dr. Michael Roizen, "Fighting Your Aging Enemies," January 15, 2006, http://www.oprah.com/article/health/wellnessandprevention/major_agers.

23. Kirsten Sauermann, Sören Jaspers, Urte Koop, and Horst Wenck, "Topically Applied Vitamin C Increases the Density of Dermal Papillae in Aged Human Skin," *BMC Dermatology*, published online September 29, 2004, http://www.ncbi.nlm.nih.gov:80/pmc/articles/PMC522805/.

24. Paula Begoun, "Vitamin C," *Cosmetics Ingredients Dictionary*, http://www.cosmeticscop.com/anti-aging-superstars-a-list-healthy-young-looking-skin.aspx#vitamin-c.

25. "Vitamin C for Wrinkles and Skin Aging," Smart Skin Care, http://www.smartskincare.com/treatments/topical/vitc.html.

26. Begoun, "Vitamin C."

27. Begoun, "Vitamin C." R. Rampoldi, N. Macedo, W. Alallon, and J. Sanguimetti, "Topical Vitamin E and Ultraviolet Radiation on Human Skin," *Medicina Cutánea Ibero-Latino-Americana*, 1990, 18 (4): 269–272; and J. C. Murray, J. A. Burch, R. D. Streilein, M. A. Iannacchione, R. P. Hall, and S. R. Pinnell, "A Topical Antioxidant Solution Containing Vitamins C and E Stabilized by Ferulic Acid Provides Protection for Human Skin Against Damage Caused by Ultraviolet Irradiation," *Journal of the American Academy of Dermatology*, September 2008, 59 (3): 418–425.

28. L. S. Baumann and J. Spencer, "The Effects of Topical Vitamin E on the Cosmetic Appearance of Scars," *Dermatologic Surgery*, April 1999, 25 (4): 311–315.

29. Begoun, "Vitamin C."

30. Paula Begoun, "Pomegranate," *Cosmetics Ingredients Dictionary*, http://www.cosmeticscop.com/anti-aging-superstars-b-list-supporting-role.aspx#pomegranate.

31. S. K. Katiyar, N. Ahmad, and H. Mukhtar, "Green Tea and Skin," *Archives for Dermatological Research*, August 2000, 136 (8): 989–994.

32. http://www.oprah.com/article/style/makeovers/skin_skinbody_nutrients/5.

33. Paula Begoun, "Coenzyme $Q_{10}$," *Cosmetics Ingredients Dictionary*, http://www.cosmeticscop.com/ingredient_dictionary.aspx?lid=500.

34. PAN Pesticides Database—Chemicals, "All-trans Retinoic Acid," http://www.pesticideinfo.org/Detail_Chemical.jsp?Rec_Id=PC42142.

35. Paula Begoun, "Retinol," *Cosmetics Ingredients Dictionary*, http://www.cosmeticscop.com/ingredient_dictionary.aspx?lid=530.

36. Paula Begoun, "Dimethylaminoethanol (DMAE)," *Cosmetics Ingredients Dictionary*, http://www.cosmeticscop.com/ingredient_dictionary.aspx?lid=502.

37. Sue Chung, "DMAE, Cell Death and Anti-Wrinkle Creams," Health Central, May 7, 2007, http://www.healthcentral.com/skin-cancer/c/115/9293/dmae-cell-death; and Anne Harding, "'Instant Face Lift' Chemical DMAE Damages Skin Cells," Reuters online, April 18, 2007, http://www.reuters.com/article/healthNews/idUSCOL85568520070418.

38. "Material Safety Data Sheet: Dimethylaminoethanol," June 15, 2006, Electron Microscopy Sciences online, http://www.emsdiasum.com/microscopy/technical/msds/13300.pdf.

39. J. R. Kaczvinsky, C. E. Griffiths, M. S. Schnicker, and J. Li, "Efficacy of Anti-Aging Products for Periorbital Wrinkles as Measured by 3-D Imaging," *Journal of Cosmetic Dermatology*, September 2009, 8 (3): 228–233.

40. "Do Peptides in Skin Care Products Work?" The Dermatology Blog, June 23, 2008, http://thedermblog.com/2008/06/23/do-peptides-in-skin-care-products-work/.

41. Paula Begoun, "Peptides," *Cosmetics Ingredients Dictionary*, http://www.cosmeticscop.com/ingredient_dictionary.aspx?lid=526.

42. A. Kawada, N. Konishi, N. Olso, S. Kawara, and A. Date, "Evaluation of Anti-Wrinkle Effects of a Novel Cosmetic Containing Niacinamide," *Journal of Dermatology*, October 2008, 35 (10): 637–642.

43. "Question: Is hyaluronic acid absorbable by the skin (topical)?" Real-Self, http://www.realself.com/question/is-hyaluronic-acid-absorbable-skin-topical-ive-read; and "About Hyaluronic Acid (HA)," http://www.hyalogic.com/about_hyaluronic_acid.htm.

44. "Dr. Perricone's Top 10 Super Supplements—# 6—Conjugated Linoleic

Acid," Daily Perricone, January 18, 2009, http://www.dailyperricone.com/2009/01/dr-perricone's-top-10-super-supplements-6-conjugated-linoleic-acid/.

45. R. S. Herbst, "Review of Epidermal Growth Factor Receptor Biology," *International Journal of Radiation Oncology, Biology, Physics*, 2004, 59 (2): 21–26.

46. C. Montecucco and J. Molgó, "Botulinal Neurotoxins: Revival of an Old Killer," *Current Opinion in Pharmacology*, June 2005, 5 (3): 274–279; Frank J. Erbguth, "Historical Notes on Botulism, *Clostridium Botulinum*, Botulinum Toxin, and the Idea of the Therapeutic Use of the Toxin," *Movement Disorders*, March 9, 2004, 19 (58): 52–56; and Jeremy Sobel, "Food Safety," *Clinical Infectious Diseases*, published online August 29, 2005, http://www.journals.uchicago.edu/doi/abs/10.1086/444507.

47. Natasha Singer, "FDA Orders Warning Label for Botox," *New York Times*, April 30, 2009.

48. Sandy Walsh, "FDA Gives Update on Botulinum Toxin Safety Warnings; Established Names of Drugs Changed," FDA News & Events, August 3, 2009, http://www.fda.gov/NewsEvents/Newsroom/PressAnnouncements/ucm175013.htm.

49. "FDA Warns About Fat-Melting Injections," http://www.msnbc.msn.com/id/27783564/ns/health-skin_and_beauty/.

50. Paula Begoun, "'Filling In' the Wrinkles," http://www.cosmeticscop.com/skin-care-facts-filling-wrinkles.aspx?filter=itemtype%3acontent.

51. "Wrinkle Relief: Injectable Cosmetic Fillers," FDA for Consumers, http://www.fda.gov/ForConsumers/ConsumerUpdates/ucm049349.htm.

52. Nora Isaacs, "Hold the Chemicals, Bring on the Needles," *New York Times*, December 13, 2007.

53. Jasmin Malik Chua, "Get a Natural Face-Lift with Face Yoga," Planet Green, March 31, 2008, http://planetgreen.discovery.com/fashion-beauty/get-a-natural-facelift.html.

## CHAPTER 6. YOUR MAKEUP

1. "Bismuth Oxychloride: Do We Really Need It?" The Green Beauty Guide, October 16, 2008, http://thegreenbeautyguide.com/?p=162.

2. Paula Begoun, "Bare Escentuals," http://www.cosmeticscop.com/brand_review.aspx?tid=178&brand=Bare+Escentuals.

3. "Nano Titanium Dioxide," Environmental Working Group's Skin Deep Cosmetic Safety Database, http://www.cosmeticsdatabase.com/ingredient.php?ingred06=726566.

4. Rita Johnson, "Lipstick," C&EN, published online July 12, 1999, http://pubs.acs.org/cen/whatstuff/stuff/7728scit2.html.

5. "Madder, Cochineal, Saffron, and Woad: Cactus Family (Cactaceae)," Wayne's Word, http://waynesword.palomar.edu/ecoph3.htm#cochineal.

6. Amy Butler Greenfield, *A Perfect Red: Empire, Espionage, and the Quest for the Color of Desire* (New York: HarperCollins, 2005).

7. "Cochineal," Reference.com, http://www.reference.com/browse/wiki/Cochineal.

8. "A Poison Kiss: The Problem of Lead in Lipstick," Campaign for Safe Cosmetics, October 2007, http://www.safecosmetics.org/downloads/A%20Poison%20Kiss_report.pdf.

9. "FDA Study: Lead Levels in Lipstick Much Higher than Previously Reported," Reuters online, http://www.reuters.com/article/pressRelease/idUS170678+01-Sep-2009+PRN20090901; and Abby Ellin, "A Simple Smooch or a Toxic Smack?" *New York Times*, May 27, 2009.

10. "Butylated Hydroxyanisole (BHA)," National Toxicology Program, http://ntp.niehs.nih.gov/ntp/roc/eleventh/profiles/s027bha.pdf.

11. N. Ito, S. Fukushima, and H. Tsuda, "Carcinogenicity and Modification of the Carcinogenic Response by BHA, BHT, and Other Antioxidants," *Critical Reviews in Toxicology*, 1985, 15 (2), 109–150.

12. Elson M. Haas and Buck Levin, *Staying Healthy with Nutrition: The Complete Guide to Diet and Nutritional Medicine* (Berkeley, CA: Celestial Arts, 2006).

13. Amelia Hill, "Make-Up Kit Holds Hidden Danger of Cancer," *The Observer*, April 7, 2002.

14. Hezreen Abdul Rashid, "Kohl for the Eyes," Urban Muslim Women, September 22, 2008.

## CHAPTER 7. YOUR BODY

1. H. S. Brown, D. R. Bishop, and C. A. Rowan, "The Role of Skin Absorption as a Route of Exposure for Volatile Organic Compounds (VOCs) in Drinking Water," *American Journal of Public Health*, May 1984.

2. Paula Begoun, "Proppylene Glycol," Paula's Choice, http://www.cosmeticscop.com/skin-care-facts-propylene-glycol-msds-concerns.aspx.

3. Propylene Glycol Material Safety Data Sheet," http://www.sciencelab.com/xMSDS-Propylene_glycol-9927239.

4. Winter, *A Consumer's Dictionary of Cosmetics Ingredients*.

5. Marisa Belger, "Want a Fresh, Green Deodorant?" MSNBC.com, http://www.msnbc.msn.com/id/21208797/.

6. "Product Safety Assessment: Propylene Glycol," Dow, http://www.dow.com/productsafety/finder/prog.htm.

7. Jerry Kronenberg, "Is Your Sunscreen Safe?" *Boston Herald*, June 18, 2007.

8. Antonia M. Calafat, Lee-Yang Wong, Xiaoyun Ye, John A. Reidy, and Larry L. Needham, "Concentrations of the Sunscreen Agent Benzophenone-3 in Residents of the United States: National Health and Nutrition Examination Survey 2003–2004," *Environmental Health Perspectives*, March 2008, 116 (7): 893–897.

9. Kim Painter, "Your Health: Sunscreen Isn't Just About SPF," *USA Today*, May 31, 2009.

10. Ker Than, "Swimmers' Sunscreen Killing Off Coral," *National Geographic*, January 29, 2009.

11. "Aluminum," Health Canada Environmental and Workplace Health, November 1998, http://www.hc-sc.gc.ca/ewh-semt/pubs/water-eau/aluminum/references-bibliographiques-eng.php.

12. P. D. Darbre, A. A. Aljarrah, W. R. Miller, N. G. Coldhan, M. J. Sauer, and G. S. Pope, "Concentrations of Parabens in Human Breast Tissue," *Journal of Applied Toxicology*, January–February 2004, 24 (1): 5–13.

13. P. D. Darbre, "Aluminium, Antiperspirants, and Breast Cancer," *Journal of Inorganic Biochemistry*, September 2005, 99 (9): 1912–1919.

14. "Parabens," FDA-Cosmetics, http://www.fda.gov/Cosmetics/Product andIngredientSafety/SelectedCosmeticIngredients/ucm128042.htm.

15. Belger, "Want a Fresh, Green Deodorant?"

16. Tabitha Morgan, "Bronze Age Perfume 'Discovered,'" *BBC News*, March 19, 2005.

17. Ibid.; and Chandler Burr, "L'Heir du Temps," *T Magazine, New York Times*, Spring 2008; and Gabriel, *The Green Beauty Guide*, 319.

18. Gabriel, *The Green Beauty Guide*, 319.

19. "The Chanel No. 5 Story," *Independent*, October 15, 2008.

20. "Making Sense of Scents," http://users.lmi.net/wilworks/ehnmsofs.htm.

21. Winter, *A Consumer's Dictionary of Cosmetic Ingredients*, 519; and "Toluene," U.S. Environmental Protection Agency Hazard Summary, April 1992, revised January 2000, http://www.epa.gov/ttn/atw/hlthef/toluene.html.

22. International Programme on Chemical Safety, "Mineral Oil," *INCHEM*, Joint FAO/WHO Expert Committee on Food Additivies, http://www.inchem.org/documents/jecfa/jecmono/v10je08.htm; and Y. Zhao, A. Krishnadasan, N. Kennedy, H. Morgenstern, and B. Ritz, "Estimated Effects of Solvents and Mineral Oils on Cancer Incidence and Mortality in a Cohort of Aerospace Workers," *American Journal of Industrial Medicine*, October 2005.

23. Gabriel, *The Green Beauty Guide*.

24. "Improper Use of Skin Numbing Products Can Be Deadly," FDA, January 2009, http://www.fda.gov/ForConsumers/ConsumerUpdates/ucm095147.htm.

25. "Stretch Marks," DermNet, http://dermnetnz.org/dermal-infiltrative/striae.html.

26. "How to Eliminate Stretch Marks," *Marie Claire*, http://www.marieclaire.com/hair-beauty/how-to/tips/stretch-marks.

27. "Oz on Call," *The Oprah Winfrey Show*, February 13, 2007, http://www.oprah.com/slideshow/oprahshow/oprahshow1_ss_20070213/2.

28. Paula, Begoun, "Caffeine," Cosmetic Ingredient Dictionary, http://www.cosmeticscop.com/dictionary_term.aspx?tid=957&lid=500&term=caffeine; and M. V. R. Velasco, C. N. T. Tsugmi, G. M. Machado-Santelli, V. O. Consiglieri, T. M. Kaneko, and A. R. Baby, "Effects of Caffeine and Siloxanetriol Alginate Caffeine, as Anticellulite Agents, on Fatty Tissue: Histological Evaluation," *Journal of Cosmetic Dermatology*, March 2008, 7 (1): 23–29.

29. M. S. Pires-de-Campos, G. R. Leonardi, M. Chorilli, R. C. Spadari-Bratfisch, M. L. Polacow, and D. M. Grassi-Kassisse, "The Effect of Topical Caffeine on the Morphology of Swine Hypodermis as Measured by Ultrasound," *Journal of Cosmetic Dermatology*, September 2008.

30. Paula Begoun, "Special Report—Caution Cellulite: Bumpy Road Ahead," http://www.cosmeticscop.com/skin-care-facts-cellulite-myths-facts-cellulite-myths-facts-produce-reviews-options-treatments.aspx.

31. Ibid.

32. "Thigh Creams," FDA, February 24, 2000, http://www.fda.gov/Cosmetics/ProductandIngredientSafety/ProductInformation/ucm127641.htm.

33. "How Do Sunless-Tanning Products Work?" Howstuffworks, http://science.howstuffworks.com/question639.htm.

34. K. Jung, M. Seifert, T. Herrling, and J. Fuchs, "UV-Generated Free Radicals (FR) in Skin: Their Prevention by Sunscreens and Their Induction by Self-Tanning Agents," *Spectrochim Acta Mol Biomol Spectros*, May 2008, 65 (5): 1423–1428.

35. Rebecca Ruiz, "Why You Should Be Getting More Sun," Forbes online, http://health.msn.com/health-topics/articlepage.aspx?cp-documentid=100238070&.

36. Dermatologists Can Help Separate Fact from Fiction for Sun Exposure, Sunscreen, and Vitamin D," American Academy of Dermatology press release, November 10, 2009, http://www.aad.org/public/sun/smart.html.

## CHAPTER 8. YOUR NAILS

1. Robert A. Schwartz, "Clubbing of the Nails," June 12, 2009, http://emedicine.medscape.com/article/1105946-overview.

2. Andrew Weil, "Worried About White Spots on Fingernails?" February 11, 2005, http://www.drweil.com/drw/u/QAA350576/white-spots-on-fingernails. html.

3. "Nails," Children, Youth, and Women's Health Service Kids' Health, http:// www.cyh.com/HealthTopics/HealthTopicDetailsKids.aspx?p=335&np=152&id =2486.

4. William Gottlieb, ed., *The Doctors Book of Home Remedies: Thousands of Tips and Technques Anyone Can Use to Heal Everyday Health Problems* (New York: Bantam, 1991).

5. "Nail Care Products," U.S. Food and Drug Administration, http://www. fda.gov/Cosmetics/ProductandIngredientSafety/ProductInformation/ucm 127068.htm.

6. Louise G. Parks, Joe S. Ostby, Christy R. Lambright, Barbara D. Abbott, Gary R. Klinefelter, Norman J. Borlow, and Earl Gray Jr., "The Plasticizer Diethylhexyl Phthalate Induces Malformations by Decreasing Fetal Testosterone Synthesis During Sexual Differentiation in the Male Rat," *Toxicological Sciences*, August 11, 2000, 58: 339–348.

7. "Formaldehyde and Cancer Risk," National Cancer Institute, http://www. cancer.gov/cancertopics/factsheet/risk/formaldehyde.

8. "What Is Household Hazardous Waste?" Los Angeles County Department of Public Works, http://ladpw.org/epd/hhw/.

9. Ibid.

10. "Nail Care Products," U.S. Food and Drug Administration.

11. From a letter from the CEO, March 15, 2007 (on file).

12. From interview notes with Rebecca Sutton at EWG, June 17, 2009.

13. "Acrylic Acid," U.S. Environmental Protection Agency, http://www.epa. gov/ttn/atw/hlthef/acrylica.html.

14. "Nail Care Products," U.S. Food and Drug Administration.

15. Ibid.; and Cosmetic Ingredient Review Expert Panel, "Final Report on the Safety Assessment of Methoxyisopropanol and Methozyisopropyl Acetate as Used in Cosmetics," *International Journal of Toxicology*, 2008, 27 (2): 25–39.

16. "Acetone," National Library of Medicine's Tox Town, http://toxtown. nlm.nih.gov/text_version/chemicals.php?id=1.

17. Toxicological Profile for Acetone, May 1994, U.S. Agency for Toxic Substances and Disease Registry, http://www.atsdr.cdc.gov/toxprofiles/phs21.html.

18. Ibid.

19. "Personal Care Products Conducts Nationwide Recall of Non-Acetone Nail Polish Remover Because of Possible Health Risk," U.S. Food and Drug

Administration Press Release, April 29, 2009, http://www.fda.gov/Safety/ Recalls/ucm143437.htm.

20. http://www.cvs.com/CVSApp/catalog/shop_product_detail.jsp;jsession id=Sw2LKKKb7l0QJf6ppvDWZjllFnWTWnXTBllZy6YN26lhtk2h2ptc!28109407 ?filterBy=&skuId=235630&productId=235630&navAction=push&navCount =1&no_new_crumb=true.

21. Bernardita Policarpio, "Skin Lightening and Depigmenting Agents," October 26, 2009, http://emedicine.medscape.com/article/1068091-overview.

22. Gottlieb, *The Doctors Book of Home Remedies*.

23. Ibid.


## CHAPTER 9. YOUR DIET

1. Barry Sears, *The Anti-Inflammation Zone: Reversing the Silent Epidemic That's Destroying Our Health* (New York: Regan Books, 2005).

2. Tanya Edwards, "Fighting Inflammation with Fish Oil," in Ask the Experts, *Cleveland Clinic Magazine*, Winter 2007, 4 (1): 40.

3. "Exercise May Help Decrease Inflammation in Skin Tissue," Science Daily, January 17, 2008, http://www.cosmeticsandtoiletries.com/research/ biology/13877737.html.

4. Andrew Weil, "Anti-Inflammatory Diet Tips," http://www.drweil.com/ drw/u/ART02012/anti-inflammatory-diet.

5. Jacqueline Stenson, "Does What You Eat Affect Your Skin? Some Foods and Supplements May Cause Problems," MSNBC.com, December 11, 2003, http://www.msnbc.msn.com/id/3076467/.

6. James Norman, "Diabetes: What Is Insulin?" EndocrineWeb.com, http:// www.endocrineweb.com/diabetes/2insulin.html.

7. Nicholas Perricone, *The Clear Skin Prescription: The Perricone Program to Eliminate Problem Skin* (New York: HarperCollins, 2004), 36.

8. Andrew Weil, *Spontaneous Healing: How to Discover and Embrace Your Body's Natural Ability to Heal Itself* (New York: Ballantine Books, 2000), 145.

9. "The Protein SRF Keeps the Skin Healthy," ScienceDaily, April 2, 2009, http://www.sciencedaily.com/releases/2009/03/090324213527.htm.

10. Bryan Walsh, "Meat: Making Global Warming Worse," Time.com, September 10, 2008, http://www.time.com/time/health/article/0,8599,1839995,00. html.

11. "Health Risks and Benefits of Alcohol Consumption," *Alcohol Research & Health*, 2000, 24 (1), 5–9.

12. "White Tea Could Keep You Healthy and Looking Young," ScienceDaily, August 14, 2009, http://www.sciencedaily.com/releases/2009/08/090810085312.htm.

13. Andrew Price, "Buying Bottled Water: Daft or Clever?" Good Magazine blog, August 1, 2007, http://www.good.is/post/buying-bottled-water-daft-or-clever/.

14. Perricone, *The Clear Skin Prescription*, 59.

15. John Cannell, "How to Get Enough Vitamin D," The Vitamin D Council, http://www.vitamindcouncil.org/.

16. Roland Staud, "Vitamin D: More Than Just Affecting Calcium and Bone," *Current Rheumatology Reports*, September 2005, 7 (5): 356–364.

17. Gretchen Reynolds, "Can Vitamin D Improve Your Athletic Performance?" *New York Times* blog, September 23, 2009, http://well.blogs.nytimes.com/2009/09/23/phys-ed-can-vitamin-d-improve-your-athletic-performance/?scp=1&sq=health%20skin%20inflammation&st=cse.

18. Wendy Leonard, "Can Omega-3s Help Fight Asthma?" Revolution Health Group, September 12, 2006, http://www.revolutionhealth.com/healthy-living/vitamins-dietary-supplements/popular-supplements/omega-3/can-omega-3s-help-fight-asthma.

19. James Kat, *The Truth About Beauty: Transform Your Looks and Your Life from the Inside Out* (New York: Atria Books, 2003), 249.

20. Ibid., 183.

21. Dirk Smillie, "A Headache for Dr. Oz," Forbes.com, June 16, 2009, http://www.forbes.com/2009/06/15/mehmet-oz-oprah-business-media-resveratrol.html.

22. Ibid.

## CHAPTER 10. YOUR LIFESTYLE

1. "The Effects of Stress," Oprah.com, November 14, 2007, http://www.oprah.com/article/oprahradio/rsmith/rsmith_20071114; and "New Research Links Social Stress to Harmful Fat Deposits, Heart Disease," Breakthrough Digest Medical News, August 5, 2009, http://www.breakthroughdigest.com/heart-disease/new-research-links-social-stress-to-harmful-fat-deposits-heart-disease/.

2. "Poll: Stress Squeezes 4 in 10 Americans: Workers, Parents, Those Under 50 Most Stressed," CBS News Health, January 30, 2007, http://www.cbsnews.com/stories/2007/01/30/health/webmd/main2414493.shtml?source=RSSattr=Health_2414493.

3. Robin Marantz Henig, "Understanding the Anxious Mind," *New York Times Magazine*, September 29, 2009.

4. Doris J. Day, *One Hundred Questions and Answers about Acne* (Sudbury, MA: Jones and Bartlett Publishers, 2005).

5. Nancy K. Dess, "Tend and Befriend: Women Tend to Nurture and Men to Withdraw When Life Gets Hard," Psychology Today online, August 12, 2009, http://www.psychologytoday.com/articles/200009/tend-and-befriend.

6. Jerome M. Siegel, "Why We Sleep: The Reasons That We Sleep Are Gradually Becoming Less Enigmatic," *Scientific American*, November 2003, 5: 92–97.

7. Ibid.

8. "Americans Get Less Sleep Than 20 Years Ago," CBS News Health, February 28, 2008, http://www.cbsnews.com/stories/2008/02/28/health/webmd/main 3889430.shtml.

9. "Why Should We Have Eight Hours' Sleep?" BBC News, April 12, 2007, http://news.bbc.co.uk/2/hi/uk_news/magazine/6546209.stm.

10. Siegel, "Why We Sleep."

11. Ibid.

12. "Is Sex Good for You?" Times of India, August 22, 2004, http://timesof india.indiatimes.com/news/sunday-toi/Is-sex-good-for-you/articleshow/ 823406.cms.

13. Ibid.

14. Kerstin Uvnäs Moberg and Roberta Francis, *The Oxytocin Factor: Tapping the Hormone of Calm, Love, and Healing* (Boston: Da Capo Press, 2003).

15. Robin Wallace, "Healthy Love Life Leads to Well-Being," FoxNews.com, February 15, 2005, http://www.foxnews.com/story/0,2933,147453,00.html.

16. Ibid.

17. Andrew Weil, *Breathing: The Master Key to Self-Healing* (Louisville, CO: Sounds True, 2005).

18. Susan Gage, "Scientists Study Links Between Brain, Meditation," OregonLive.com, June 19, 2008, http://www.oregonlive.com/health/index.ssf/2008/ 06/scientists_study_links_between.html.

19. Ibid.

20. Ray Sahelian, "Oxytocin Hormone Benefits and Side Effects," ray sahelian.com, http://www.raysahelian.com/oxytocin.html.

21. Erin Olivo, "Energy Medicine," Oprah.com, January 15, 2006, http:// www.oprah.com/article/health/wellnessandprevention/energy_basics.

22. P. Silverstein, "Smoking and Wound Healing," *American Journal of Medicine*, July 15 1992, 93 (1A): 225–245.

23.   http://www.plasticsurgery.org/Documents/Media/Twins-PRS-Study-2009.pdf.

24. Tara Parker-Pope, "Social Smoking Takes a Lasting Toll," *New York Times* Health blog, October 8, 2008, http://well.blogs.nytimes.com/2008/10/08/occasional-smoking-takes-a-lasting-toll/.

25. "*Yoga Journal* Releases 2008 'Yoga in America' Market Study," http://www.reuters.com/article/pressRelease/idUS147936+26-Feb-2008+PRN 20080226.

26. L. Cohen, C. Warneke, R. T. Fouladi, M. A. Rodriguez, A. Chaoul-Reich, "Psychological Adjustment and Sleep Quality in a Randomized Trial of the Effects of a Tibetan Yoga Intervention in Patients with Lymphoma," *Cancer*, May 2004, 15, 100 (10): 2253–2260.

27. Kate Hanley, "Improve Your Sex Life with Yoga," Gaiam Life, http://life.gaiam.com/gaiam/p/Improve-Your-Sex-Life-with-Yoga.html.

28. Michelle Stewardson, "Calm Cure: Yogic Breathing and Gentle Poses Help Keep the Body's Lymph Fluid Circulating," yogajournal.com, http://www.yogajournal.com/health/1690.

29. "The Endocrine System (Glands) and Yoga," ABC-of-Yoga.com, http://www.abc-of-yoga.com/health/glands.asp.

## AFTERWORD

1. The Estée Lauder Companies Inc., press release, *Business Wire*, January 28, 2010.

2. "Proposition 65," Office of Environmental Health Hazard Assessment, http://oehha.ca.gov/prop65/p65faq.html.

3. Ibid.

4. "Minnesota Bans Adding Mercury to Cosmetics," CBSNews.com, December 14, 2007, http://www.cbsnews.com/stories/2007/12/14/health/main3618048.shtml.

# Acknowledgments

To say we feel grateful for the opportunity to write about this subject—and write about it together—doesn't quite cut it. Of course, the idea might never have materialized without that fated blowout, and so we extend our heartfelt thanks to a certain West Hollywood salon, and to the mean hairdresser who made us cry.

We could not have made sense of the science without the countless experts who so generously gave us their time: Dr. Michael DiBartolomeis, Dr. Mitchell A. Kline, Dr. Leslie Baumann, Dr. Earl Gray, Dr. Joseph Schwarcz, Dr. Dave Hobson, Dr. Doris Day, Dr. Alexander Rivkin, Dr. Ladan Mostaghimi, Thu Quach, Dr. Peggy Reynolds, Dr. Rebecca Sutton, Stacy Malkan, Paula Simpson, and Betty Bridges. We are also thankful to Jessa Blades, Karen Behnke, Spirit Demerson, Evan Healy, Tara Kee, John Masters, Josie Maran, Horst Rechelbacher, Elisha Reverby, and Rose-Marie Swift for sharing their insight and candor; to David Biello, Graham Fidler, Peter Rubin, Matt Smith, Bryan Walsh, Jaime Wolf, and Aviva Yael for their early guidance; and to the GOOD team, and Morgan Clendaniel and Zach Frechette for their friendship and support throughout this whole process.

Thanks to Sloan Harris for leading us to Tina Wexler at ICM, who has been a most gracious steward, taking us through this process gently and with many laughs. We're also grateful to our editor Katie McHugh at DaCapo Lifelong, who let us write the book we wanted but made it better, and to Georgia Feldman, Alex Camlin, David Steinberger, and the entire Perseus Books Group family for their support, as well as to Lori Hobkirk at the Book Factory and to proofreader Sandy Chapman.

We were lucky to have exceptional sounding boards along the way. Thank you to the many friends who helped us brainstorm, read rough drafts, experimented on their faces, and listened to our rants: Carol Cho, Carolina Crespo, Jessica de Ruiter, Lesley Desaulniers, Michelle Diamond, Diana Gitelman, Thomas Golianopoulos, Jermaine Hall, Emily Hamphire, Kathleen Jensen, Debra Lawrence, Simone Leblanc, Mark Mann, Aska Matsumiya and the L.A. Ladies Choir, Adam Matthews, Caitlin McKenna, Amanda Millner-Fairbanks, Jeb Reed, Erika Sasson, Nathaniel Schachter, Katie Schad, Amy Schwartz, Marina Sharpe, Anna Singer, Mark Slutsky, Emily Southwood, Nikhil Swaminathan, Mathew Swenson, Jacob Tierney, Datwon Thomas, Bonsu Thompson, Matt Thompson, Ethan Tobman, Liza Vadnai, Robbie Vroom, and Kim Waldron. Last but not least, thanks to two very patient guys: Nate Scott and Steve Thrush.

Finally, we are so grateful to our families: our wonder siblings Denis O'Connor, Shannon O'Connor, and Nicola Spunt; our parents Anne and Dennis O'Connor, and Louise and Ronald Spunt; and to Patty and Emmett Francoeur, Maeve, and Conall Francoeur, and Christina Kalcevich.

In the loving memory of Barbara Singer and to those who share her spirit.

We thank you all, and we thank each other.

# Index